T0233998

LIBERATION BY OPPRESSION

Books by Thomas Szasz

Pain and Pleasure
The Myth of Mental Illness
Law, Liberty, and Psychiatry
Psychiatric Justice
The Ethics of Psychoanalysis
The Manufacture of Madness
Ideology and Insanity
The Age of Madness (ed.)
The Second Sin
Ceremonial Chemistry
Heresies
Karl Kraus and the Soul Doctors
Schizophrenia
Psychiatric Slavery
The Theology of Medicine
The Myth of Psychotherapy
Sex by Prescription
The Therapeutic State
Insanity
The Untamed Tongue
Our Right to Drugs
A Lexicon of Lunacy
Cruel Compassion
The Meaning of Mind
Fatal Freedom
Pharmacracy
Liberation by Oppression
Words to the Wise
Faith in Freedom

LIBERATION BY OPPRESSION

A Comparative Study of
Slavery and Psychiatry

THOMAS SZASZ

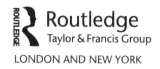

Routledge
Taylor & Francis Group

LONDON AND NEW YORK

First published 2002 by Transaction Publishers

Published 2017 by Routledge
2 Park Square, Milton Park, Abingdon, Oxon OX14 4RN
711 Third Avenue, New York, NY 10017, USA

Routledge is an imprint of the Taylor & Francis Group, an informa business

Library of Congress Catalog Number: 2001052503

Library of Congress Cataloging-in-Publication Data

Szasz, Thomas Stephen, 1920-
    Liberation by oppression : a comparative study of slavery and psychiatry / Thomas Szasz.
        p. cm.
    Includes bibliographical references and index.
    ISBN 0-7658-0540-5 (alk. paper)
        1. Psychiatric hospitals—United States. 2. Involuntary treatment—Moral and ethical aspects. 3. Slavery—United States—History. 4. Mentally ill—Treatment—History. 5. Socially handicapped—Mental health services. 6. Psychiatric ethics. 7. Paternalism—Moral and ethical aspects. 8. Social control. 9. Antipsychiatry. I. Title.

RC443 .S98   2002
616.89—dc21   2001052503

ISBN 13: 978-0-7658-0540-9 (pbk)

Tell me, who was it who first declared, proclaiming it to the whole world, that a man does evil only because he does not know his real interests, and if he is enlightened and has his eyes opened to his own best and normal interests, man will cease to do evil and at once become virtuous and noble, because when he is enlightened and understands what will really benefit him he will see his own best interest in virtue, and since it is well known that no man can knowingly act against his best interests, consequently he will inevitably, so to speak, begin to do good. Oh, what a baby! Oh, what a pure, innocent child!

Fyodor Dostoyevsky
Notes from Underground[1]

Contents

Acknowledgments

No man is an island, and no book is, strictly speaking, the creation of a single individual. I am deeply indebted to my family, friends, colleagues, and fans for conversations, criticisms, suggestions, and sources; for reading and correcting the manuscript; and, last but not least, for supporting a point of view thought wrongheaded or worse by the cognoscenti.

I wish to thank especially Peter Uva, librarian at the SUNY Upstate Medical University at Syracuse, for his generous and wise help, year after year, book after book; also, my brother George, daughter Margot, Keith Hoeller, Charles Howard, Alice Michtom, Jeffrey Schaler, Mira de Vries, and Roger Yanow. I hope I have expressed my gratitude to them in person better than I could in these few words.

Grateful acknowledgment is made for permission to reprint the following copyright material:

Alexander, G. J. and Scheflin, A. W., "Lobotomy," in *Law and Mental Disorder* (Durham, NC: Carolina Academic Press, 1998). Copyright 1998 by Carolina Academic Press. Used by permission of the publisher.

Jon Dougherty, "Testing the faith: Student sues college for psychiatric abuse, sent to mental ward after he objected to play depicting Jesus as homosexual," *WorldNetDaily*, January 5, 2001, http:// www.scotsman.com/cfm/home/email_a_friend_part2.cfm, © 2001 WorldNetDaily.com. Reprinted with permission of the Internet newspaper *WorldNetDaily.com*.

Maggie Farley, "Mental illness by mandate," *Los Angles Times*, February 10, 2000. © 2000, Los Angeles Times. Reprinted with permission.

Hundley, T., "'Last prisoner of WWII' looks for a memory: Held 56 years in Russia, Hungarian recalls little," *Chicago Tribune*, September 7, 2000. © 2000, Chicago Tribune. Reprinted with permission.

Preface

> We have seen the mere distinction of colour made in the most enlight-
> ened period of time, a ground of the most oppressive dominion ever
> exercised by man over man.
>
> —*James Madison (1768-1849)*[1]

> Yes, disguise it as we may, we do keep...*in a sort of slavery* a multitude of
> unfortunates who sigh for liberty and to whom it would be sweet.
>
> —*Samuel Gridley Howe, M.D. (1801-1876)*[2]

Comparing psychiatry with slavery—implying that they are similar kinds of institutions and human relations—may, at first glance,
seem bizarre, even obscene. Psychiatry is good. Slavery is evil. But
it is not that simple.

James M. McPherson, professor of American history at Princeton,
begins his magisterial work, *Battle Cry of Freedom*, with these words:
"Both sides of the American Civil War professed to be fighting for
freedom."[3] Supporters of the Confederacy believed they were for
"freedom," by which they meant "State sovereignty": they sought to
liberate the Confederacy from the shackles of a tyrannical, national
state—the Union. Opponents of the Confederacy also believed
they were for "freedom," by which they meant preserving the
Union against secession and, if they were abolitionists, freeing
the slaves. Supporters of what I call *psychiatric slavery* also claim
they are for freedom: they seek to liberate the mental patient from
the shackles of his illness. But here the similarity ends: unlike the
numbers of people who supported the opponents of the Confederacy during the Civil War, few support the opponents of psychiatric
slavery.

On March 12, 1861, Alexander Hamilton Stephens (1812-1883),
vice president of the Confederate States, delivered a speech in Sa-
vannah, Georgia that included the following: "[The Confederacy]
rests upon the great truth that the negro is not equal to the white
man: that slavery, subordination to the superior race, is his natural

and moral condition. This, our new Government, is the first, in the history of the world, based on this great physical, philosophical, and moral truth."[4]

The justification for contemporary psychiatric coercion strongly parallels Stephens's statement. To paraphrase: our society rests upon the great truth that the mental patient is not the equal of the psychiatrist, that his subordination to the scientific doctrine of mental health is his medical and moral duty. Even if we grant that many persons considered mentally ill are less capable of meeting their needs for shelter, food, and human relations than are psychiatrists, it does not follow that mental patients ought to be under the forcible domination of psychiatrists. The only thing that follows is that some mental patients might benefit from access to asylums—places of sustenance and refuge from the demands of society that provide these patients with their basic needs, but without depriving them of their basic rights.

We can study psychiatry by examining its ostensible subject matter, mental illness, or by examining what its practitioners, psychiatrists, do. Although these two approaches seem to be complementary, they are not. In fact, they are mutually antagonistic. Why? Because the idea of mental illness implicitly requires and justifies psychiatric coercions and excuses.[5] Until we recognize this simple truth, there can be no real progress in understanding the phenomena we call "mental diseases" and no genuine reform of the psychiatric practices we call "psychiatric treatments."

Psychiatry began as mad-doctoring and soon became a medical specialty, called "neuropsychiatry," seemingly based on neuropathology. Today, psychiatry is based on politics: the state proclaims that psychiatry is a branch of medicine and that mental diseases are brain diseases—because the mind is a product of the brain.[6]

More than forty years have passed since I declared, in *The Myth of Mental Illness*, my psychiatric agnosticism and opposition to forcible psychiatric "treatment." In this book, I show that psychiatric theory is about behaviors, not diseases, and that psychiatric practice is about oppression/liberation, not the use or abuse of a branch of medicine.

During most of the twentieth century, psychiatry was a house divided—one part concerned with the control of involuntary mental patients, another part with contractual relations between consenting adults. This is no longer true. For all practical purposes, the house of psychiatry is now undivided. During the last few decades, the American people—politicians, psychiatrists, physicians, medical researchers, lawyers, journalists, the public—have embraced what they regard as a new, value-free science of biological psychiatry. The radical differences between the coercive character of mental hospital practices and the consensual character of private psychotherapeutic practices are denied.

The truth is that coercive psychiatry serves the interests of the coercers, and that contractual psychiatry serves the interests of the contracting parties. Acknowledging this fact is taboo, intellectually, professionally, and politically. The mandatory view is that science is leading us to the recognition of increasing numbers of discrete mental diseases, each of which requires treatment with specific drugs; and also to the recognition of increasing numbers of lawless acts as the manifestations of mental diseases, all of which require treatment with psychiatric detention and psychiatric drugs. In other words, we are advancing toward the view that good behaviors are choices attributable to free will, meriting praise; and that bad behaviors are the symptoms of brain diseases, exempting the "patient" from blame, often mandating psychiatric incarceration.

The human rights violations of chattel slavery, the Inquisition, National Socialism, and Communism have been well documented. My goal is to show that psychiatry—as the oppression of the patient by the psychiatrist, defined and justified as the patient's liberation from an illness that robs him of freedom and responsibility—belongs in this pantheon of man's inhumanity to man.

Introduction: Perilous Rescues

The madman is not the man who has lost his reason. The madman is the man who has lost everything except his reason.
—*Gilbert K. Chesteron (1874-1936)*[1]

Sometimes there are judgments at which one arrives that one hesitates to state publicly, out of respect for deeply held beliefs and prejudices.
—*Frank S. Meyer (1909-1972)*[2]

For centuries, people believed that in addition to benefiting the community, forcibly curing the soul of the heretic was good for the heretic, forcibly enslaving the Negro was good for the slave, and forcibly treating the insane was good for the mental patient. A single idea animates each of these protective-persecutory ideologies: that saving people from themselves is good not only for the community but for the coerced person as well.

With respect to liberating the insane by oppressing him, we have, during the past few decades, gone from bad to worse. Until recently, the space where mental patients could be forcibly treated was limited to the confines of the insane asylum or mental hospital. Today, there is no longer any legal boundary between the mental hospital and society: regardless of where a person may be located, the psychiatrist, assisted by the judge, can impose diagnosis and treatment on him, against his will.

In *The Manufacture of Madness: A Comparative Study of the Inquisition and the Mental Health Movement* (1970), I presented a systematic account of the similarities between past coercive religious practices and present coercive psychiatric practices. In this book, I offer a systematic account of the similarities between chattel slavery and psychiatric slavery, the term I use to describe psychiatric interventions imposed on persons by force. Inasmuch as the Inquisition forms the template for all subsequent Western ideologies of saving people from themselves, I shall begin with a brief review of that often misunderstood institution.

1

The Inquisition: Protecting People from Error

Religious beliefs and practices are inherently both public and private, social and individual, uniform and diverse. From its formal founding in the fourth century, the Catholic Church has had a hierarchical structure, with a central bureaucracy. This is why, for Catholicism—unlike Buddhism or Judaism—the diversity of religious beliefs became heresy and hence a "social problem" that had to be dealt with. There is far too little appreciation that tolerance for deviance—with respect to religious belief, sexual behavior, drug use, and so forth—prevents behavioral diversity from becoming a "problem" that requires an ideology and social machinery to "explain" and "solve" it.

The word "heresy" is derived from the Greek *hairesis*, which originally meant an act of choosing. "As so used," explains the *Encyclopaedia Britannica*, "the term was neutral, but once appropriated by Christianity it began to convey a note of disapproval. This was because the Church from the start regarded itself as the custodian of a divinely imparted revelation... Thus, any interpretation which differed from the official one was necessarily 'heretical,' in the new, pejorative sense."[3]

Orthodoxy implies heterodoxy. The history of Christianity is, in part, the history of heresy—religious "error," committed by individuals or sects, "corrected" by the True Church. Initially, heretics—such as the Arians, Manicheans, Albigensi, and Donatists—were suppressed by bishops and their secular allies. In the twelfth century, Church councils began to require secular rulers to prosecute heretics. The founding of the Inquisition is usually credited to Pope Gregory IX (1145-1241; Pope 1227-1241) who, in February, 1231, "enacted a law for Rome that heretics condemned by an ecclesiastical court should be delivered to the secular power to receive their 'due punishment.' This 'due punishment' was death by fire for the obstinate and imprisonment for life for the penitent."[4] The Spanish Inquisition was formally established in 1478. We should note, in this connection, that the word "inquisition," like the word "heresy," began life as a term of approbation and gradually changed into a term of condemnation. The word derives from the Latin *inquirere*, which means to look into or inquire. Originally, it referred to a special ecclesiastical institution for combating and suppressing heresy—a "war" deemed to serve the best interests of both the heretic and the community.[5]

The similarities between Inquisitorial and psychiatric procedures are dramatic and obvious: the person accused of heresy was presumed guilty, had to testify against himself, and the more fervently he denied being a heretic, the more obstinately heretical he was deemed to be. He had no right to question his accusers. "It was acceptable to take testimony from criminals, persons of bad reputation, excommunicated people, and heretics. The accused did not have right to counsel, and blood relationship did not exempt one from the duty to testify against the accused. Sentences could not be appealed... Penalties went from visits to churches, pilgrimages, and wearing the cross of infamy to imprisonment...and death by burning at the stake, [which] was carried out by the secular authorities...accompanied by the confiscation of all the accused's property."[6]

In 1542, Pope Paul III established a permanent congregation, staffed with cardinals and other officials, whose task was to defend the integrity of the faith and proscribe errors and false doctrines. This body, the Congregation of the Holy Office, now called the Congregation for the Doctrine of the Faith, part of the Roman Curia, became the supervisory body of local Inquisitions. It was this body that placed Copernicus's *De Revolutionibus Orbium Coelestium* on the *Index of Forbidden Books* and tried Galileo.[7]

The Catholic Encyclopedia rightly emphasizes that "Moderns experience difficulty in understanding this institution, because they have, to no small extent, lost sight of two facts. On the one hand they have ceased to grasp religious belief as something objective, as the gift of God, and therefore outside the realm of free private judgment; on the other they no longer see in the Church a society perfect and sovereign, based substantially on a pure and authentic Revelation, whose most important duty must naturally be to retain unsullied this original deposit of faith. Before the religious revolution of the sixteenth century, these views were still common to all Christians; *that orthodoxy should be maintained at any cost seemed self-evident.*"[8]

Truth and Intolerance

The idea that possessing the truth obligates one to tolerate error is a modern, scientific idea. Its scope is still largely limited to the hard sciences, attested to by the now fashionable intolerance in the social sciences, politics, the media, and everyday life called "political correctness."

The Church was viewed as having been established by Christ, as a perfect society. It followed that it must be empowered to make laws and inflict penalties for their violation. Thus, heresy—viewed as the violation of the laws of the Church, striking at her very life, the unity of belief—"was a crime which secular rulers were bound in duty to punish. It was regarded as worse than any other crime, even that of high treason."[9]

Religious intolerance was not peculiar to Catholicism. It was, and is, the natural accompaniment of deep religious conviction. Allied with power, its inexorable consequence is religious persecution. After the Reformation, religious persecutions became intensified, Calvin's Geneva becoming the seat of the Protestant "inquisition."

Psychiatric intolerance is one of the pillars of the therapeutic state. Its trinity—psychiatric diagnosis, psychiatric treatment, and psychiatric incarceration—is a mask for justifying coercion as care. Rejecting psychiatric treatment and rejecting life (i.e. attempting suicide) are psychiatric heresies, punishable by psychiatric incarceration and involuntary psychiatric treatment. Opposition to coercive psychiatric suicide prevention is reflexively dismissed as so lacking in compassion as to be unworthy of consideration.[10]

The repentant Catholic heretic often embraced the faith more ardently than his persecutor, if for no other reason than to demonstrate his reliability and insure his own safety. The repentant psychiatric heretic does the same. Commenting on the Surgeon General's declaration of war on mental illness, Kay Redfield Jamison, professor of psychiatry at Johns Hopkins Medical School, declared: "As someone who studies, treats and suffers from a severe mental illness—manic depression, I commend the surgeon general for his excellent, thoughtful and fair report on mental illness."[11] Not satisfied with endorsing involuntary mental hospitalization and involuntary electric shock treatment, Jamison asserts that "the distinction between voluntary and involuntary commitment is misleading and arbitrary."[12]

We have made great progress since the Inquisition: we have chemicals that cure our heretics, and we regard our cured heretics as the most knowledgeable and scientific of inquisitors. I maintain that Richard Feynman was right: "Who are the witch doctors? Psychoanalysts and psychiatrists, of course... We live in an unscientific age... Science is the belief in the ignorance of the experts."[13] We believe in the infallibility of the psychiatric expert.

Psychiatric Slavery

Psychiatric slavery—that is, confining individuals in madhouses— began in the seventeenth century, grew in the eighteenth, and became an accepted social custom in the nineteenth century. Because the practice entails depriving law-abiding individuals of liberty, it requires moral and legal justification. The history of psychiatry, especially regarding its relation to law, is largely the story of the mutating justifications for psychiatric incarceration. The metamorphosis of one criterion for commitment into another is typically called "psychiatric reform." It is nothing of the kind. The bottom line of the psychiatric balance sheet is fixed: individuals deemed insane are stigmatized, incarcerated, and forcibly "treated." For more than forty years, I have maintained that psychiatric reforms are exercises in prettifying plantations. *Slavery cannot be reformed—it can only be abolished.* As long as the idea of mental illness connotes dangerousness and legitimizes psychiatric power exercised through preventive psychiatric detention, psychiatric slavery cannot be abolished. (Although the idea of mental illness implicitly imparts legitimacy to the exercise of psychiatric power, it does not, per se, prevent the abolition of psychiatric slavery. Some abolitionists believed in the racial inferiority of the Negro. Some ex-patients believe in mental illness but oppose psychiatric coercion.[14])

Power is the ability to compel obedience. Its sources are force from above, and dependency from below. By force I mean the legal and/or physical ability to deprive another person of life, liberty, or property. By dependency I mean the desire or need for others as protectors or providers. To distinguish between coercive and noncoercive means of securing obedience, we must distinguish between force and persuasion, violence and authority. Alfred North Whitehead put it thus: "[T]he intercourse between individuals and between social groups takes one of these two forms, force and persuasion. Commerce is the great example of intercourse by way of persuasion. War, slavery, and governmental compulsion exemplify the reign of force."[15] When Voltaire exclaimed, *"Écrazez l'infame!"* he was using the word *"l'infame"* to refer to the power of the Church to torture and kill, not to its power to misinform or mislead.

Like the inquisitor, the contemporary psychiatrist has a hard time distinguishing between repudiating the Other's (false) ideas but tolerating him, and persecuting the Other to help him see the "truth." In the zealot's eyes, tolerance of psychiatric heresy is tantamount to a declaration of war on Psychiatry. Why? Because, unlike standard medical practice, which rests on cooperation, standard psychiatric practice rests on coercion. This is what seems to make opposition to psychiatric coercion the same as opposition to psychiatry *in toto*. Abolitionists opposed only the legally sanctioned coercion of black persons. I oppose only the legally sanctioned coercion of persons with psychiatric diagnoses. Psychiatric relations between informed consenting adults ought to be a matter of private contract.

Psychiatric Slavery and the Therapeutic State

Psychiatric slavery is the oldest and most characteristic feature of the therapeutic state, which, in turn, is the modern, secular incarnation of the theocratic state. Each is a species of political absolutism: one based on the pharmacratic rights of medical protectors, the other on the divine rights of royal protectors. Since its inception, the power and prestige of psychiatric slavery have steadily grown and the coercive psychiatric system is now an integral and respected part of every modern society. Why, then, do I oppose it? Because I believe that the coercive control of bad behavior ought to be a moral and political, not a medical or therapeutic, function; and that the state ought to punish only illegal behavior and ought to do so only by criminal sanctions. In short, I oppose psychiatric slavery because I believe it is inimical to individual liberty and responsibility, to the rule of law, and to the very existence of a free society.

However, most people see psychiatry not as enslavement to a destructive ideology, but as liberation from a dangerous illness; they accept the claims that psychiatry is a medical science and psychiatric interventions are scientifically valid medical treatments of real diseases. They do not see that the lot of psychiatric slaves is as miserable as ever, partly because they do not want to see it, and partly because making diagnoses and prescribing medications make psychiatrists look like real doctors, who are perceived as intrinsically benevolent. A study of patients' attitudes toward physicians revealed that "Mostly patients trust doctors."[16]

Formerly, mental patients were restrained physically, without the pretense of treatment; now, they are restrained chemically, and this pharmacological restraint masquerades as treatment. Formerly, the madman incarcerated in the madhouse was perceived as an incompetent person with an incurable illness; now, he is perceived as a dangerous patient suffering from a treatable illness, but lacking insight into his condition and hence requiring treatment against his will. "People will not accept medication if they don't think they're sick," explains E. Fuller Torrey, head of the Treatment Advocacy Center in Arlington, Virginia. "That's why people with severe mental illness must be treated involuntarily."[17]

Overwhelming support for psychiatric slavery, by public policy and public opinion alike, deprives the critic of a forum for effective dissent, regardless of the absurdity of the claim he criticizes. "It is axiomatic in medicine," declares Stephen Rachlin, professor of psychiatry at Columbia University College of Physicians and Surgeons, "that the patient is hardly in the best position to prescribe his own treatment."[18] Rachlin equates the medical patient's right to reject treatment prescribed for him by a physician with his "right" to decide and dictate treatment for himself to be administered by a physician. This, of course, is nonsense. But Rachlin's distortion enables him to ask: "How, then can we say that he [the mental patient] is able to make an informed choice as to whether or not treatment is indicated? In my experience, the psychiatric inpatient refusing treatment does so for reasons related to his psychosis and thought disorder...if freedom is to be more than just another word, the right to refuse treatment is one right too many."[19]

Can anyone have too much freedom? Not if we use the word as Lord Acton used it: "The center and supreme object of liberty is the reign of conscience... Liberty is the condition which makes it easy for conscience to govern."[20] Were psychiatrists to acknowledge Acton's views on liberty, their consciences would disable them from doing their work. Unhampered by such an impediment, psychiatrists can indulge their zeal to make the patient happy by giving him treatments, even against his will. They are unaware of Acton's warning: "If happiness is the end of society, then liberty is superfluous. It does not make men happy."[21]

The transformation of our image of psychiatry from what it had been prior to World War II to what it is today is due in part to the Holocaust and the horrors of the war. In the aftermath of these events, virtually everyone became a self-styled champion of "human rights." For blacks and women, the result was salutary: they gained genuine legal rights. For mental patients, the result was disastrous: they gained the "right" to be mental patients which, in practice, meant the duty to submit to cruel and unusual punishments defined as treatments. Coercive psychiatric practices are now more common, affect more persons, and are believed to be better justified than they have ever been. The modern mental patient is the beneficiary of a host of new laws "empowering" him with a gift-list of rights, such as the right to a lawyer, the right to treatment, the right to be confined in the least restrictive setting, and so forth. Instead of liberating the mental patient from domination by the coercive psychiatrist, these measures have reinforced the legitimacy of psychiatric oppression as medical care. The following example illustrates how lawyers, judges, and psychiatrists now collaborate in practicing psychiatric slavery.[22]

A man, considered *competent and not dangerous*, is committed to a mental hospital. Psychiatrists want him to take neuroleptic drugs. He refuses. His captors petition the court to authorize involuntary treatment. The judges order the patient-prisoner to be drugged against his will. The court ruled:

We recognize that this holding is inconsistent with our statement that "the state may not act in a parens patriae relationship to a mental hospital patient unless the patient has been adjudicated incompetent." We no longer adhere to that absolutist position... Under the more modern view...*a person's involuntary commitment to a hospital due to a mental illness does not even raise a presumption that the patient is incompetent*... When a court finds by clear and convincing evidence that a patient lacks the capacity to give or withhold informed consent regarding treatment, then the state's interest in caring for its citizen overrides the patient's interest in refusing treatment. When, in addition, the court also finds by clear and convincing evidence that the benefits of the antipsychotic medication outweigh the side effects, and that there is no less intrusive treatment that will be as effective in treating the illness, then it may issue an order permitting forced medication of the patient."[23]

The Curse of the Curability of Mental Illness

We have come a long way since the days when insanity was considered incurable. Considering insanity curable has made the insane person's situation worse, not better. As long as the psychiatrist believed that insanity was incurable, the patients were, to some extent, protected from the psychiatrist's *furor therapeuticus*. Conversely, the more obsessed the psychiatrist becomes with his power to defeat mental illness, the more enraged he becomes by the patients' rejection of treatment. Thus, some of the worst abuses of psychiatry have been committed in the name of psychiatric treatment, such as insulin coma therapy, electric shock treatment, and lobotomy. Today, we can add psychotropic drugs to that list.

When chattel slavery was the law, people were not interested in the lessons the history of slavery held for them. Today, people are not interested in the lessons the history of psychiatry hold for them; instead, they cling to self-flattering falsehoods, such as the belief that in the past, without effective treatments, insane persons were condemned to suffer the dire consequences of their untreated illness. This is not true.

Two hundred years ago, Sir George Baker (1722-1809), President of the Royal College of Physicians, observed: "Nor let us immediately despair...that, because the patient cannot be relieved by art, he therefore cannot be relieved at all. For Madness...oftentimes ceases spontaneously."[24] Similarly, Philippe Pinel (1745-1826), the father of French psychiatry, stated: "We likewise know, that a certain permanent cure may be obtained by what the French call the method of expectation, which consists solely in delivering up the maniac to the efforts of unassisted nature."[25] In 1900, a psychiatrist writing in the *Journal of the American Medical Association* reported that "66.7 percent of the commitments [to the Government Hospital for the Insane] recovered in an average period of 3.9 months."[26] This is a better outcome than any produced by coerced drugging today.

Accepting that a disease is incurable need not signify defeat and helplessness. On the contrary, it can be the incentive for genuine compassion and true helpfulness. Accepting that, at some point, some bodily illnesses are incurable has led to the creation of the modern hospice movement. Hospice patients are not expected to make use of the most up-to-date treatments and are not required to live as long as possible. Acceptance that mental diseases are incurable—because they are not diseases—could similarly be an incentive for genuine compassion and true helpfulness. In particular, it could lead—if we really wanted to serve the self-defined interests of the denominated patient (rather than his family or society)—to the creation of a true asylum: an institution where a person could safely seek shelter and sustenance, would not be expected to submit to any treatment or change his behavior, and would not be expelled from it against his will (except for criminal behavior or behavior violating the rules of conduct set forth by the providers of the asylum).

If the true asylum is a place where persons defined as "different" by the majority, or the state, are offered protection from those intent on depriving them of their right to be different, then it must be a place free of coercion: people must be able to enter and leave it at will. A clear concept of the asylum helps us to understand its mirror images: the mental hospital and the concentration camp. Contrary to common belief, the concentration camp is neither a National Socialist nor a Communist invention; instead, it is a late nineteenth-century Spanish-colonial invention, originating in Cuba. What makes concentration camps different from other places of confinement? "When we speak of concentration camps," suggests journalist Anne Applebaum, "we generally mean camps for people who have been *imprisoned not for what they have done but for who they are*."[27] Exactly the same is true for mental hospitals.[28]

Unfortunately, the advent of mad-doctoring was accompanied by a perversion of the word "asylum," which Samuel Johnson defined as "a place out of which he that has fled to it, may not be taken."[29] When we speak of the United States as giving asylum to the immigrant, we mean that, here, the immigrant is free from coercion based on who he is. This may be true for the immigrant, but is not true for the mental patient. And this was never true of the insane asylum, which, from the start, combined the functions of the asylum—protecting the inmates by locking out society—with the functions of the penitentiary—protecting society by locking up the "patient." In 1838, in his influential treatise tellingly titled *Total Abolition of Personal Restraint in the Treatment of the Insane,* Robert Gardiner Hill (1811-1878)—a Scottish physician and the owner of several insane asylums—lamented: "Let it be indeed a Refuge from distress; an Asylum, not in name, but in deed and in truth—a place where the sufferer may be shielded from injury and insult—where his feelings may not be uselessly wounded, nor his innocent wishes wantonly thwarted."[30] There would have been no need to say this had the word "asylum"—in "insane asylum"—not already been hijacked and turned into signifying the opposite of its root meaning.

The asylum functions of the state mental hospitals, unsatisfactory and indeed unacceptable as they were, disappeared soon after the advent of the mass drugging and deinstitutionalization of mental patients. The leading, albeit fictitious, selling point of these "reforms" was that they rendered long-term hospitalization for mental illness unnecessary. As a result, in the West today, virtually the only place of refuge for the individual who wants to escape the demands of society is suicide.[31]

Deinstitutionalization—a euphemism for the forcible eviction of the mental patient from the mental hospital—was followed by laws mandating "outpatient commitment"—another euphemism, for forcing the patient to ingest psychiatric drugs while "living in the community." This sequence of events resembles the Jim Crow laws after the "liberation" of slaves by the Civil War and the Thirteenth Amendment. In each case, members of the stigmatized and oppressed class are nominally liberated from their shackles, making them free and equal in theory, only to be re-oppressed by a new set of laws and policies, making them once again unfree and unequal in practice.

Before concluding these introductory remarks, I want to acknowledge that the comparison of psychiatric slavery with chattel slavery fails in one important respect. From the earliest days of chattel slavery in America, many prominent members of the oppressor class felt a deep sense of guilt for the practice, which they recognized as a profound moral offense against the Negro slave, whose humanity was self-evident. The Declaration of Independence spelled the doom of chattel slavery. More specifically, the deeds and words of the first three American presidents signified the recognition, among the leaders of the land, that slavery was, simply, wrong. George Washington provided for the emancipation of his slaves in his will. John Adams rejected owning slaves and declared: "Every measure of prudence ought to be assumed for the eventual total extirpation of slavery in the United States." Jefferson famously wrote, "I tremble for my country when I think that God is just," and stated that "it was among his first wishes to see some plan adopted by which slavery in this country might be abolished by law."[32]

This is not the way American presidents or leading politicians, physicians, priests, and pundits speak about psychiatric slavery today. Accordingly, popular sentiment overwhelmingly favors incarcerating innocent persons (civil commitment) and excusing guilty persons (and incarcerating them also, called "the insanity defense"), both state-police interventions masquerading as humane and scientific treatments. Many mental patients and ex-mental patients, though dissatisfied with one or another aspect of psychiatric practices, proclaim their belief in mental illness and reject the abolition of psychiatric slavery. Virtually everyone believes that psychiatric coercions and excuses are "liberal," "progressive" social practices and "moral advances." Over what? Over what is fatuously called "unjustly punishing innocent persons," as if a voluntary system of curing souls were not an option for those who obey the law, and as if a humane system of fines and prison sentences were not the proper penalties for those who break the law.

Neither in the United States nor anywhere else in the world have a significant number of persons expressed interest in securing freedom from coerced psychiatric meddling. Quite the contrary. Most Americans sincerely believe that expanding the scope of psychiatric slavery would benefit the country, just as most slaveholders in the early 1800s sincerely believed that expanding chattel slavery would benefit it. This is not difficult to understand, provided we are willing to recognize the self-flattering ideology of "helping"—Christianizing and curing, as the case may be—that sustained chattel slavery and now sustains psychiatric slavery.

Much as slaveholders liked to view themselves as rescuing the Negro from savagery, psychiatrists like to view themselves as rescuing the involuntary patient from insanity. "It seems to me that if there is a right to drown," declares Darold A. Treffert, a forensic psychiatrist in Wisconsin, "there must also be a right to be rescued."[33] Treffert ignores not only the right to be left alone, but also that having a right to be rescued entails someone else's obligation to rescue. He assumes—as do most Americans—that the obligation to rescue mental patients is the God-given job of the psychiatrist. Thus are psychiatrist and mental patient entwined in a deathly embrace, drowning together in a sea of diagnoses and drugs.

Chattel slavery was the original sin of the American ideal of individual liberty, a sin the nation has still been unable fully to expiate. Psychiatric slavery, I shall argue, is the Achilles heel of that ideal, a fatal flaw that may yet transform the American dream into an American nightmare.

1

Psychiatric Slavery: Legal Fiction and the Rhetoric of Therapeutic Oppression

[Slavery is] a moral, social, and political blessing... [It is] the most humane of relations of labor to capital which can permanently subsist between them.

—Jefferson Davis (1808-1889)[1]

I think it is a very hard case for a man to be locked up in an asylum and kept there; you may call it anything you like, but it is a prison.

—Sir James Coxe (1877)[2]

In two earlier books—*Psychiatric Slavery* (1977) and *Insanity: The Idea and Its Consequences* (1987)—I discussed the similarities between the rhetoric of coercive paternalistic therapeutism characteristic of both involuntary servitude and involuntary psychiatry. In this chapter, I reconsider the parallels between these two institutions and show that the practice of psychiatric slavery is, just as the practice of chattel slavery was, incompatible with a moral commitment to personal responsibility and individual liberty.

The Experience of Losing Liberty

One of my most vivid childhood memories is being forced, when I was six, to go to school. I wanted to stay home. Why did I have to go to school? Because, I was told, all children my age went to school, and because it was good for me. It didn't feel that way. It felt like punishment.

Later, I learned that people who did bad things were locked up in bad places; that there were two kinds of bad people—criminals and crazies; and two kinds of bad places where they were locked up—prisons and mental hospitals. Thus, for me, the most obvious thing about mental hospitals has always been that they are *very* bad places. The persons locked up say they are bad and, to make matters worse, the persons who lock them up say they are good places, and that they are especially good for those who are locked up.

Adults who are labeled "mentally ill" are not children. Most of them have not been convicted of a crime. Mental illnesses, whatever they are, are not contagious. Why, then, are persons with psychiatric diagnoses deprived of liberty? According to the authorities, mental patients are ill and dangerous; they need to be institutionalized for their own welfare and for the protection of society. This explanation never made sense to me. By the time I was an adolescent, I concluded that people declared to be crazy are incarcerated because they embarrass their family; that removing them to insane asylums serves the interests of their relatives and other members of society; and, most importantly, that inquiring into the justification for locking up mad people is taboo. Crazy people belong in madhouses. Only a crazy person would ask, *why?*

After I became a physician and decided to turn my attention to psychiatric problems, the involuntary legal status of the mental hospital patient became, for me, *the* defining characteristic of psychiatry as a medical discipline, as (then) distinguished from psychoanalysis, which entailed only listening and speaking, and prohibited touching the patient except for shaking hands.

Why do psychiatrists lock up innocent mental patients and declare some criminals "not guilty"? Why do psychiatrists say that mental patients are "hospitalized" and "treated," instead of saying they are "deprived of liberty," or are "incarcerated," or are "deprived of responsibility and treated as if they were infants or incompetents?" Why do people call persons incarcerated in insane asylums "sick" and say they have a brain disease, even though pathologists cannot find any post-mortem evidence of such disease? Why do lawyers insist that legal punishment ought to be reserved for mentally healthy persons and that the psychiatric coercion of individuals called "mentally ill" is not punishment? In short, why can't we relate to these persons as our moral equals? Why can't we regard them as we regard ourselves, as responsible moral agents or persons?

Well aware that asking such questions is taboo, an offense not only against psychiatry but also against conventional wisdom, I waited until I completed my psychiatric and psychoanalytic training before systematically addressing, and challenging, the practice of involuntary mental hospitalization. I was not surprised to discover, in the 1950s, when I was gathering materials for what became *The Myth of Mental Illness* and *Law, Liberty, and Psychiatry*—that most psychiatric textbooks were silent on the subject of coercion.[3] Psychiatrists pretended that mental patients are admitted to state mental hospitals the same way that medical patients are admitted to regular hospitals. The few psychiatrists who did acknowledge the existence of commitment laws claimed that such laws ought to place little, if any, restrictions on the psychiatrist's professional discretion to determine who qualifies for psychiatric deprivation of liberty, because legal limits on the psychiatrist's powers to commit would be obstacles to good patient care. In 1948, the Group for the Advancement of Psychiatry—a prestigious post-war organization of prominent psychiatrists whose aim was to improve the public image of psychiatry—stated: "The Committee believes that all statutes should delete the term 'commitment'... 'Insanity' and 'lunacy' should be replaced by the term 'mental illness'."[4] In 1958, the authors of a leading textbook of psychiatry declared: "The psychiatrist urges that the dignity of the patient be respected and that the obstacles to his admission be no greater than those experienced by the physically ill."[5] Many psychiatrists still share this view.

The proposal of these post-World War II "reformers" quickly gained professional and popular acceptance. Now, fifty years later, both groups are unhappy with the results, and are intensifying their efforts to medicalize behavior and transform psychiatric coercion into help. They are like George Santayana's fanatics, who redouble their efforts after they lose sight of their goal. For three hundred years, mad-doctors and psychiatrists maintained that mental illnesses are brain diseases and that incarcerating mental patients is a form of hospitalization. During this time, not a single officially accredited medical or scientific body rejected this claim as false and immoral. Notwithstanding the glaring evidence to the contrary, psychiatrists keep reassuring themselves and the public that madness is a real medical malady and that madhouses are true hospitals. How are we to understand this history and this situation? The best way to do so is by seriously scrutinizing the power of the psychiatrist to imprison and the status of the mental patient as prisoner—in short, by taking seriously the similarities between slavery and psychiatry.

Chattel Slavery and Psychiatric Slavery

The *Encyclopaedia Britannica* defines slavery as "the social sanctioning of involuntary servitude imposed by one person or group upon another."[6] I define psychiatric slavery as the social sanctioning of involuntary psychiatric "diagnosis" and "treatment" imposed by one person or group upon another person or group.

Chattel slavery is one of the oldest social institutions. Psychiatric slavery is one of the youngest. The basic element shared by both is the use of force by one person to make another do something against his will. As long as an oppressive practice is customary, it is, by definition, acceptable; it may even be viewed as altruistic: the coercer is perceived as caring for, educating, or treating the coerced. "A long habit of not thinking a thing *wrong*," observed Tom Paine, "gives it a superficial appearance of being *right*, and raises at first a formidable outcry in defense of custom."[7] Once the legitimacy of the practice is seriously challenged and people begin to have qualms about it, the practice tends to be perceived as abusive—with the coercer seen as exploiting, victimizing, "raping" the coerced, or, in more modern terms, the coercer depriving the coerced of his "human rights."

In ancient Greece and Rome, the head of the household—father and husband—had absolute authority over his wives, children, and slaves. This is the source of the association of slavery with the notions of patriarchy, paternalism, domesticity, dependency, altruism, and caring, and, for a long time, its non-association with race. The master coerced, controlled, *and* cared for his family and his slaves. The psychiatrist is expected to, and is legally authorized to, coerce, control, *and* care for his patients.

Like the family, slavery appears to be a universal institution or type of social arrangement, based partly on power, and partly on authority, rooted in the belief that persons who possess physical, intellectual and/or financial power ought to have the right to control others. Greek and Roman customs and laws, as well as the great monotheistic religions, are steeped in and reflect this mind set. Parents have unlimited powers over their children, masters over their slaves, God over all living creatures. For millennia, slavery—serfdom, vassalage—was an institution considered indispensable for the proper functioning of society. Indeed, the practice of slavery is by no means extinct today.[8]

Although the liberation of the biblical Jews from slavery is celebrated in Exodus, there is no condemnation of the practice in the Old or New Testaments or the Koran. Jews, Christians, and Mohammedans alike owned and traded slaves. So, too, did blacks and whites. In fact, one of the largest slaveholders in nineteenth-century South Carolina was a black man, named April Ellison.[9] In the Christian West, the Scriptures and the Church became the foremost legitimizers of slavery. These are familiar facts. I mention them to underscore that, throughout most of history, people viewed slavery as a socially necessary institution and that this perception was shared by both masters and slaves. The same is now true for psychiatric slavery.

The Anatomy of Psychiatric Slavery

All modern societies recognize the legally authenticated domination of persons called "mental patients" by agents of the state called "psychiatrists" as an indispensable social practice and morally praiseworthy medical institution. None recognize this practice as a form of systematic oppression. Until its final days, the same was true for slavery. According to the *Encyclopaedia Britannica,* "Although slavery in its various forms was an almost universal institution, or rather because of that, little or no opposition was raised against it. There were, of course, denunciations of its excesses, at times, and attempts to remedy abuses, but the existence of the institution was not questioned until the beginning of the modern antislavery movement at the end of the 16th century and the beginning of the 17th century."[10] David Brion Davis—professor of history at Yale and a distinguished student of slavery—underscores this point: "Today, it is difficult to understand why slavery was accepted from prebiblical times in virtually every culture and not seriously challenged until the late 1700's. But the institution was so basic that genuine antislavery attitudes required a profound shift in moral perception. This meant fundamental religious and philosophic changes in views of human abilities, responsibilities and rights."[11]

No one contests that coercive police practices serve the interests of the community and not the interests of the persons detained by the police. However, few concede that coercive psychiatric practices serve the interests of the community and not the interests of persons detained by psychiatrists. This denial legitimizes the consequences of psychiatry's two paradigmatic procedures, civil commitment and the insanity defense. Civil commitment is a legal procedure for depriving innocent persons of liberty by confining them in mental institutions against their will. The insanity defense is a legal procedure for excusing guilty persons of responsibility for their crimes and then incarcerating them in mental institutions.[12] For three hundred years coercion and the threat of coercion have framed the context of the psychiatrist's daily work. Modern societies regard psychiatric slavery as a morally praiseworthy institution, a hallmark of humanism informed by science.

Children and other dependents are forced to interact with countless persons whom they might prefer to avoid, for example, siblings, parents, teachers, schoolmates, counselors, psychologists, and priests. In contrast, adults, in a free society, enjoy the basic right of associating with others or avoiding them. To be sure, there are some persons with whom adults may sometimes be *forced* to associate, such as policemen and agents of the Internal Revenue Service. The psychiatrist belongs on this list, with this important difference: People do not view the policeman who arrests a robber as the criminal's benefactor, but they do view, or are supposed to view, the psychiatrist who diagnoses and detains a depressed person as the detainee's benefactor. This legally and socially authenticated *definition of an adversarial relationship as a therapeutic relationship* renders the person with a psychiatric diagnosis utterly helpless and defenseless. Psychiatrists have long had a veritable love affair with coercion as benevolence. The modern psychiatrist's love for using force to "help" patients knows no bounds.

Everything people do to satisfy an appetite can be done to excess. Before the twentieth century, it never occurred to people to regard drunkenness as a disease. Today, "alcoholism" is viewed not merely as a disease but as a disease that justifies involuntary psychiatric treatment. "For addicts," writes Sally Satel, who teaches psychiatry at Yale and works in a methadone clinic in Washington, D.C., "force is the best medicine... Voluntary help is often not enough."[13] The task of the psychiatrist in a methadone clinic is to convert the addict from dependency on a drug the patient controls to dependency on a drug the doctor controls. It is hardly surprising that coercion is needed to accomplish this job.

Clearly, having involuntary patients is useful for psychiatrists and many others as well. To be sure, psychiatric slaves are useful in a different way than were chattel slaves. For millennia, labor was scarce and mass poverty was the norm: slave-laborers were needed to produce goods and services. Slavery was feudalism writ large. Slaves, laboring in the fields and the homes, were *producers of goods and services*; their social status, however, was that of dependents (they were the prototypical "child-workers"). Today, in advanced societies, labor is plentiful and the state is Croesus: slave-patients are needed to *produce work and jobs for others*. Psychiatric slavery is statism writ large. Psychiatric slaves, treated in hospitals, clinics, and the offices of mental health professionals, are consumers (of health care services); their social status, however, is that of dependents (they are incompetent, insane, non-responsible).

During the past several centuries, social controls based on domestic dependency and inferior social status were gradually replaced with social controls based on illness and treatment, especially mental illness and mental treatment.[14] Instead of needing coerced-submissive workers, today's masters need coerced-submissive patients (and "disabled" welfare recipients).

As involuntary servitude differs from voluntary labor, so involuntary psychiatric treatment differs from voluntary medical treatment. Slavery and psychiatric treatment rest on coercion; voluntary labor and medical treatment rest on cooperation. The psychiatrist-slaveholder views his patient as an individual deprived of moral agency by mental illness; the patient requires treatment against his will, for his own benefit. The contractual medical doctor views his patient as a moral agent, possessing the same rights and responsibilities as he does; each is free from coercion by the other, and each is responsible for his own behavior.

For millennia, slavery was legitimized by divine law, natural law, or, simply, conquest. Advocates of American chattel slavery made use of all these rationalizations and added a new one, beneficence. Slavery, as Vice President John Caldwell Calhoun (1782-1850) famously put it, was not an evil, but a "positive good... the most safe and stable basis for free institutions in the world."[15] David Brion Davis commented: "If it was a crime, as many writers asserted, to deprive Americans of their natural liberty, it was actually an act of liberation to remove Negroes from their harsh world of sin and dark superstition." A leading pro-slavery economist declared: "I cannot but think their condition is much bettered to what it was in their own Country."[16]

A Brief History of Psychiatric Slavery

Medicine may be said to have begun with sick persons seeking help from individuals to whom they attributed the ability or power to cure, such as elders of the tribe, shamans, kings, priests, physicians. That is not the way psychiatry began. Even psychiatric historians, looking through rose-colored lenses, do not claim such an origin for the practice that was called "mad-doctoring" before it became psychiatry. Quite the contrary. The very essence of what we now call "severe mental illness"—formerly called "psychotic illness"—is that the afflicted person "denies" that he is ill and rejects help. Herein lies the fundamental similarity between the slave and the involuntary mental patient: both reject the "care" imposed on them by their self-appointed benefactors.

Everyone wants to believe that one's own behavior is morally praiseworthy, especially if the individual profits from it economically and existentially. Thus, persons whose work depends on the routine use of coercion—for example, policemen, judges, Internal Revenue Service agents—believe that the force they exercise is justified because it is necessary and beneficial for society. Appropriately, the law calls this principle "police power."

A different kind of justification is called for when the persons who exercise coercion believe that their beneficiaries are the persons coerced. The paradigm case for this kind of justification of coercion is the relationship between the parent and the minor child. Appropriately, the law calls this principle "parens patriae" (the state as parent).

Chattel slavery was, and psychiatric slavery is, justified by appeals to both principles. The slave was, and the insane patient is, viewed as a child-like person, requiring the care of protectors—masters/psychiatrists (parens patriae). In addition, the slave was, and the insane patient is, perceived as potentially dangerous if left at liberty; hence, his coercive care is justified by the need to protect the community (police power). These images and justifications formed, and continue to form, the basis of the profession of psychiatry.

The Association of Medical Superintendents of American Institutions for the Insane (AMSAII)—the parent of the American Psychiatric Association (APA)—was founded in 1868. Its founders believed that being incarcerated in an insane asylum—that is, in a state institution, operated by physicians paid by the state—was a right belonging to the incarcerated individual: "The Association of Medical Superintendents of American Institutions for the Insane, believing that certain relations of the insane should be regulated by statutory enactments calculated to secure their rights... recommend that the following legal provisions be adopted by every State whose existing laws do not, already, satisfactorily provide for these great ends."[17]

Samuel Gridley Howe (1801-1876), physician and social reformer, was not fooled. A year after the founding of the AMSAII, he declared: "Yes, disguise it as we may, we do keep... in a sort of slavery a multitude of unfortunates who sigh for liberty and to whom it would be sweet."[18]

In the 1880s, an Australian psychiatrist named George A. Tucker visited a number of American mental hospitals and came away with this impression:

> Cages, iron chains, handcuffs, hobbles, straps, crib beds, and fixed chairs are common modes of restraint for patients, who being afforded no means of occupation or diversion for mind or body, naturally become noisy and troublesome... In the covered hot bath, the head alone protruding, the patient is confined, unable to move, from one to twelve hours at a time, and in many instances unattended, with water at a temperature of 35 degrees Centigrade, and often with cold water dripping on the head. This, I have been gravely but rather needlessly informed, was not adopted as medical means of improving the patient, but simply to quiet and subdue him for the time being.[19]

Bizarre as it may sound, psychiatric slavery was based on the premise that persons called "mental patients" had a right to be psychiatric slaves. However, owning slaves implies that the slaveholder assumes certain obligations for housing and feeding them. As one might expect, the dismal conditions to which the enslaved mental patients were consigned soon called forth reformers, eager to prettify the plantations. In 1880, the National Association for the Protection of the Insane and the Prevention of Insanity (NAPIPI)—an early version of the National Alliance for the Mentally Ill (NAMI)—was formed. In an essay tellingly titled "Despotism in Lunatic Asylums," Norman B. Eaton, one of the founders of NAPIPI, complained:

> He [the asylum superintendent] is an autocrat—absolutely unique in this republic—supreme and irresistible alike in the domain of medicine, in the domain of business, and in the domain of discipline and punishment. He is the monarch of all he surveys, from the great palace to the hencoops, from pills to muffs and handcuffs... This unparalleled despotism—extending to all conduct, to all food, to all medicine, to all conditions of happiness, to all connections with the outer world, to all possibilities of regaining liberty— awaits those whose commitments may easily be unjust if not fraudulent, whose life is shrouded in a secrecy and seclusion unknown beyond the walls of an insane asylum.[20]

Psychiatry's modern hagiographers took care to erase the memory of the psychiatrists' crimes against humanity. In 1941, Gregory Zilboorg, author of the influential *History of Medical Psychology*, looked back at the hospital superintendents Eaton had castigated and saw only "humane and learned" men and their "unique achievement":

> In the United States the physician interested in the mentally ill devoted himself almost exclusively to hospital administration, to an almost devotional training and organization of appropriate staffs of attendants, and to the creation of a unique type of mental hospital medical superintendent—a man humane and learned, who was to be physician and guide, master and assiduous pupil. In the course of the [nineteenth] century, the theory and practice of American psychiatry was the theory and practice of institutional psychiatry, which culminated in a unique achievement.[21]

Psychiatric historians and psychiatric practitioners deny the ongoing psychiatric holocaust. Journalists and the public, fearing to appear ignorant of the widely celebrated scientific advances in psychiatry, do not challenge its diagnoses allegedly based on brain scans, and its claims for cures attributed to neuropsychopharmacological miracle drugs. How are we to explain this? Understanding the concept of legal fiction—and, specifically, its use to legitimize chattel slavery in the past, and psychiatric slavery now—goes a long way toward answering that question.

Chattel Slavery, Psychiatric Slavery, and Legal Fictions

The object of both law and psychiatry is the regulation of human behavior. Yet, neither law nor psychiatry recognizes persons *simply as* persons: The law deals with rules and procedures, psychiatry, with diagnoses, diseases, and treatments.

On October 31, 2000, the *Detroit Free Press* published a special supplement entitled "Body & Mind." The subtitle, set in extra large type, read: "Mentally ill people need treatment, but their broken brains convince them they don't." This formulation postulates that there exists in American society a group of people who need something ostensibly good for them that they do not want and refuse to accept. This is pure psychiatric propaganda.

"Of all the painful puzzles the families of seriously mentally ill people face," writes the reporter, "this is the biggest one: Why do so many refuse treatment? And if they get better on medication, why do so many stop taking it?"[22] This is a puzzle only for persons who use their eyes for something other than seeing. After all, the experts themselves insist that psychiatric drugs make crazy people non-crazy. Hence, once a crazy person has been properly medicated with such drugs and is "in remission," he should be regarded as being able to make a rational decision about his further treatment. If he stops taking his medication, shouldn't we conclude that he does so because he decides that it harms rather than helps him?

However, since the patient's psychiatrists and relatives want him to continue taking the drugs, the experts dismiss the simple explanation offered above. They maintain that the hallucinating and delusional mental patient refuses to take psychiatric drugs because his "voices" tell him he doesn't need them; and that if, after taking drugs that stop his hallucinations, the patient still refuses to take drugs, it is because he denies his illness. "Of the five million Americans every year who suffer an acute mental illness," the reporter explains, "at least 60 percent are unaware of their illness or deny they are sick. About half of the people who do get medication don't take it or stop taking it."[23]

Why do crazy people claim they are not crazy? The reporter has an explanation for that, too: "For years, doctors blamed denial of severe mental illness, which in medical shorthand is called 'poor insight,' on defensiveness, anger or stubbornness." Now we know better: "Brain researchers suspect that severe mental illness could be traced to damage in the frontal lobes of the brain, which are vital to reasoning. The phenomenon of poor insight mimics a neurological problem called anosognosia, a form of frontal lobe damage in which patients give wild explanations to divert any evidence that contradicts their old self-concept."[24]

This pretentious nonsense may sound persuasive provided the reader is ignorant about neurology and schizophrenia. Anosognosia occurs most often in stroke victims. For example, after a right hemisphere stroke, the patient may refuse to admit to weakness in his left arm. This belief—not dispelled by demonstrating to the patient that his arm is paralyzed—usually lasts only a few days after the onset of the stroke and disappears without treatment.[25] Unlike patients with schizophrenia, patients with anosognosia are neither hospitalized nor treated against their will. The false analogy between the patient diagnosed with anosognosia and the patient diagnosed with schizophrenia is typical of the deceptive rhetoric supporting psychiatric slavery.

The Masks of Law and the Masks of Psychiatry

In his important book, *Persons and Masks of the Law*, John T. Noonan, Jr.—a judge on the United States Court of Appeals, Ninth Circuit—uses the example of chattel slavery to illustrate how legal fictions may be used to deny reality. Everything he says on this subject also applies to psychiatry.

Noonan writes: "Indifference to persons in legal history and legal study is dramatically illustrated by their [legal scholars'] unconcern for a major function of Anglo-American law for three centuries, the creation and maintenance of a system in which human beings were regularly sold, bred, and distributed like beasts."[26] Ignoring the commonsense perception of the Negro as a human being, legislators, lawyers, and judges "said not a word on how the legal system made a person a non-person."[27]

Similarly, legislators, lawyers, and judges ignore how, by declaring an individual mentally ill and incarcerating him in a mental hospital, the legal system makes a person a non-person. "How," asks Noonan, "could a lawyer look upon persons as kitchen utensils?" How, we might ask, could a doctor look upon (physically healthy) persons as a bundle of dysfunctional neurons?[28] The answer, in each case, is that practical necessities require such inhumanities and justify them as humane practices. In colonial Virginia, writes Noonan, "at least half of the property cases involved the disposition of slaves. He [a judge] could not have compassion for each of them and still be a judge. His role in a slave system necessitated the use of masks... Property, applied to a person, is a perfect mask. No trace of human identity remains."[29] Schizophrenia is an equally perfect mask. Countless cases coming before judges today involve issues concerning the mental health of defendants or litigants. Neither judges nor psychiatrists can have compassion for them as individuals and still fulfill their professional duties. Everyone who makes use of mental health laws and practices—perhaps most importantly the relatives of mental patients—needs the fiction of mental illness, with its implications of disease, dangerousness, and incompetence, to help him perceive responsible adults as if they were helpless infants.

It is important to keep in mind that Noonan's use, and my use, of the term "legal fiction" rests on a kind of moral revisionism, judging past practices in terms of present values. Do the following statements assert fictions or truths?

- The Negro slave is property, not person.

- The hallucinating schizophrenic is commanded by "voices" and is not responsible for his crimes.

Such statements are fictions only in hindsight or only in the eyes of skeptics or outsiders. The United States Supreme Court, the American Bar Association, the American Medical Association, and American Psychiatric Association all have affirmed the reality of one or both of these fictions. Woe to him who—at the wrong time or in the wrong place—denies that they are the Truth.

As long as Fiction counts as Truth, discourse in acceptable language precludes not only skepticism, but plain speaking itself. Chattel slavery was intrinsic to the social structure of the newly founded United States; the integrity of the new nation depended on the acceptance of the practice and the fictions used to sustain it. Despite this, or rather because of it, the term "slavery" does not appear in the Constitution. In Article I, Section 2, stipulating the method for apportioning Representatives, slaves are referred to as "three fifths of all other Persons."[30] Similarly, words such as "madness," "insanity," "mental illness," and "addiction" do not appear in the Constitution. Nevertheless, the Supreme Court has affirmed and reaffirmed the legality and morality of both chattel slavery and psychiatric slavery. For example, in *Robinson v. California* (1962), the Court factualized the fiction of addiction as a mental illness and validated the psychiatric claim that incarceration is treatment:

> It is unlikely that any State at this moment in history would attempt to make it a criminal offense for a person to be mentally ill... The addict is a sick person. He may, of course, be confined for treatment... Cruel and unusual punishment results not from confinement but from convicting the addict of a crime... If addicts can be punished for their addiction then the insane can also be punished for their insanity. Each has a disease and each must be treated as a sick person.[31]

The assertion that "the addict is a sick person" is a calculated falsehood, illustrative of the deceit intrinsic to the legal-psychiatric fiction of mental illness. The Court calls addicts "sick" to justify their status as psychiatric slaves, just as it had called black people "chattel" to justify their status as plantation slaves.

As long as chattel slavery was the custom, it was accepted as socially beneficial. "As long as the teaching of lawgivers was accepted," writes Noonan, "slavery could not be criticized without aspersion on the goodness of wealth itself."[32] Similarly, as long as the teaching of lawgivers (about mental illness) is accepted, psychiatric slavery cannot be criticized without aspersion on the goodness of health itself. As long as physicians, jurists, and journalists accept that incarcerating persons ostensibly to stop them from killing themselves is a *bona fide* medical treatment, and that acquitting murderers as mentally ill to prevent the legal system from "punishing" them as criminals is a moral good, the foundations of psychiatric slavery will remain untouched. It is a mistake to assume that murderers are acquitted as insane to avoid their execution. Defending killers as mentally ill is equally popular in European countries where capital punishment has been abolished.

Montesquieu's (1689-1755) reflections on modern, race-based slavery are pertinent in this connection. Pondering how white men can believe that black men are not human beings, he mocked the pretension on which it rests: "It is impossible that we should suppose those people [Negro slaves] to be men, because if we should suppose them to be men, we would begin to believe that we ourselves are not Christians."[33] Similarly, it is impossible that we should suppose psychiatric slaves to be persons possessing rights and responsibilities, because if we should suppose them to be such persons, we would begin to believe that we ourselves are not lovers of liberty.

Noonan does not shirk from blaming many of the Founders, and those in the legal profession, for legitimizing and perpetuating slavery. He writes: "Without their [the lawyers'] professional craftsmanship, without their management of the metaphor, without their loyalty to the system, the enslavement by words more comprehensive than any shackles could not have been formed."[34] The founders of psychiatry aided by the legal profession have exhibited the same devotion to legitimizing and perpetuating psychiatric slavery.[35]

Shackles made of legal and psychiatric words, supported by judicial sanctions and psychiatric coercions, support an intricate web of ostensibly therapeutic excuses and coercions, formally known as psychiatry. Calling that entire system "psychiatric slavery" and insisting that the "services" it renders ought to be delivered without coercion or not at all, challenges one of our most important metaphors and social practices.

Why Psychiatry is Synonymous with Psychiatric Slavery

From the founding of madhouses in the seventeenth century until the dawn of the twentieth century, all mental hospital inmates were "certified," that is, committed by law, against their will. "Until 1881," writes Howard Zonana, professor of psychiatry at Yale, "the idea of voluntary admission for someone considered mentally ill was inconceivable."[36] As late as the 1940s, when I was a medical student in Cincinnati, there were no voluntary patients in Ohio's state hospitals.

The compound term "certifiable lunatic" points to the close connections assumed to exist between insanity and incompetence. The certifiable lunatic is viewed not only as a person incapable of knowing or representing his own best interest, but also as an orphan or unwanted child, whose care, by default, becomes the duty of the state as substitute parent (*parens patriae*). Agents of the state must house him, feed him, and control him. For centuries, people accepted, as Gregory E. Pence, a medical ethicist and professor of philosophy at the University of Alabama in Birmingham, puts it, "that the insane needed 'therapeutic justice' rather than criminal justice. Since insanity was not a crime, no legal proceedings were required to commit a person thought to be insane to an institution. It was simply assumed that the committing psychiatrist would always act in the patient's best interests."[37] The assumption that the psychiatrist-master is like a good parent who serves the best interests of his psychiatric slave, as if the patient were his own child, is a fiction essential for the integrity and survival of psychiatric slavery.

In nineteenth-century psychiatry, the view of the insane individual as a sick patient suffering from a brain disease co-existed comfortably with the view that he was a naughty child in the body of an adult. For example, Heinrich Neumann (1814-1884), a leading German psychiatrist, declared: "The mental patient must be handled like an ill-behaved child, and the measures used to correct the child can also be used to advantage with the lunatic."[38] Neumann, at least, was consistent. He also believed, as do I, that "The time has finally come for us to stop looking for the herb or salt or metal which in homeopathic or allopathic doses will cure mania, imbecility, insanity, fury or passion. They will never be found until pills are discovered which will transform a naughty child into a well-mannered child, an ignorant man into a skilled artist, a rude swain into a polished gentleman... Man's psychic activities are changed, not by medicines but by habit, training and exertion."[39]

Psychiatric practices are bound to remain controversial and problematic as long as we cannot decide how to regard mental patients, psychiatrists, and mental hospitals. Are mental patients competent adults who ought to be treated as moral agents, or incompetent wards of the state who ought to be sheltered by deprivation of liberties? Are psychiatrists regular physicians or jailers? Are psychiatric institutions hospitals or prisons?

Before slavery could be abolished, its rationalizations based on Scripture, genetics, and paternalism had to be undermined. Abolitionists accomplished that goal. Similarly, before psychiatric slavery can be abolished, its rationalizations based on disease, dangerousness, and treatment—and, most importantly, protecting the individual from himself—have to be undermined. Like the abolition of chattel slavery, the abolition of psychiatric slavery must be a collective effort. For now, psychiatric slavery is indispensable for the functioning of American society, as the case of Russell Weston illustrates.

In 1998, Weston, a man with a twenty-year history of revolving mental institutionalization and deinstitutionalization, shot and killed two police officers at the United States Capitol. Diagnosed as suffering from paranoid schizophrenia, he was declared mentally incompetent, and held, pending trial, at the Federal Correctional Institute in Butner, North Carolina. For twenty years, by word and deed, Weston had expressed his wish to not take "any psychoactive medication."[40] He had refused to take the medication prescribed at Butner. The prosecution petitioned the court to authorize doctors to drug Weston against his will. Weston's court-appointed lawyer, and some psychiatrists, opposed Weston's involuntary medication, not on the ground that he is entitled to refuse such "treatment," but on the ground that they, his self-appointed protectors, do not believe in the death penalty. The possibility of Weston's execution and its prevention by a successful insanity defense gave some psychiatrists an opportunity to pose as moralists and humanists. Others were satisfied to mouth the mantra that drugging mental patients—Weston included— serves their best interests.

In April 2001, after years of wrangling in the courts, a judge ordered Weston to be forcibly medicated; in July, the United States Court of Appeals for the District of Columbia Circuit upheld the ruling. Psychiatrist Jeffrey Metzner, chair of the APA Council on

Psychiatry and Law, agreed: "It is ethical to treat a psychotic, deteriorating individual, even if the result is that he can then stand trial. It is certainly possible that the medication may relieve the person's pain." Weston, however, did not complain of pain. Rephrasing the rhetoric of rescuing Negroes from their savage state, Metzner explained: "You do not do a person with severe psychosis any favors when you leave him untreated."[41]

With all the powers of the law, medicine, the press, and public opinion safely in their hands, the defenders of psychiatric slavery claim the moral high ground. A prominent American psychiatrist offers this explanation for why mental patients' "rights are taken from them":

> ...to aid and assist the individual, to provide means whereby the state may protect its unfortunate citizens, to furnish hospitalization so that the insane will have an opportunity for rehabilitation and readjustment into useful and happy citizens... The confinement is not intended as punishment but solely and only to provide the mentally sick with that environment which may possibly cure the disease and return them to society as useful citizens. One might wish to add that we also take into consideration the dangers to society which sometimes ensue from the actions of the mentally sick.[42]

The pro-psychiatric slavery mindset has changed little since this was written some fifty years ago. To be sure, psychiatrists no longer expect the crazy person to be useful or happy. They expect him only to "take his medication," to prove to doctors that he suffers from a "treatable illness." And the rhetoric has grown ever more sanctimonious: psychiatrists have taught lay persons to evangelize the public with the message, "Committing a loved one can be the best medicine...commitment can be an empowering process for people with mental illness."[43]

Psychiatry's elephant is still in the room, with this difference: in the past, the distinction between care and coercion, voluntary and involuntary psychiatric intervention, was a taboo subject; now, it is a nonexistent subject. With one voice, leading mental health experts and politicians declare that, in psychiatry, there is no difference between care and coercion. David Mechanic—René Dubos Professor of Behavioral Sciences at Rutgers University and one of the most prominent non-physician authorities on mental illness—explains: "It is his [the psychiatrist's] role to do his best in managing patients who come to see him either because they are experiencing pain or maladjustment in their lives or because others in the community insist on some intervention."[44] Committed mental patients do not "come to see" coercive psychiatrists; they are brought to them against the detained person's will, typically in restraints.

Mechanic's defense of psychiatric power is unqualified and shameless. "The clinician," he continues, "does not decide whether people are or are not sick but generally assumes illness of some kind."[45] The medical doctor who assumes bodily illness is called a "charlatan," not a "clinician." A clinician worth his salt does precisely what Mechanic says he does not do. So why does Mechanic make this absurd assertion? To support his argument that "the psychiatrist engaged in everyday clinical work may have very little to gain by using a disease perspective... *The problem in psychiatry is really no different from the situation in general medicine.*"[46] That is the message politicians, lawyers, journalists, and the public want to hear. That message has succeeded in silencing all efforts to distinguish between voluntary and involuntary psychiatric relations and, increasingly, even between voluntary and involuntary medical relations.[47] Having shored up the psychiatrist's credentials as benevolent physician to his prisoner-patient, Mechanic declares: "The continuation of the debate [about mental illness] has become counterproductive... Far too much discussion has been devoted to the issue as to whether psychiatric conditions are diseases."[48] This conclusion is arrogant and unwarranted: Only a few years ago, the American Psychiatric Association declared that homosexuality—for decades one of its most treasured mental diseases—is not a disease and removed it from its *Diagnostic and Statistical Manual of Mental Disorders.*

Because today any condition considered a disease is of interest to the state, it is of the utmost practical importance what is, and what is not, officially classified as disease. When the church was allied with the state, rejecting certain religious teachings was defined as heresy, and priests had the power to burn heretics at the stake. When church and state were separated, rejecting religious teachings ceased to be defined as heresy, and priests lost their power to persecute persons who disagreed with them. It is only because psychiatry is allied with the state that deviance from psychiatric norms is defined as disease and psychiatrists have the power to coerce mental patients. If psychiatry and the state were separated, deviance from psychiatric norms would cease to be considered diseases and psychiatrists would lose their power to coerce persons who disagree with them.

The Original Sin of Psychiatry

The subject matter of psychiatry is conflict, not illness. The physician who decides to become a psychiatrist chooses to become a party to conflict. I use the phrase "psychiatry's original sin" to refer to the psychiatrist's *choice* to conflate coercion with care and thus defy Jesus' injunction "Render therefore unto Caesar the things which are Caesar's; and unto God the things that are God's."[49]

In fact, psychiatry is a branch of the law, concerned with preventing and punishing crime and deviance. In practice, psychiatry is a branch of medicine, concerned with diagnosing and treating disease. In one of his roles, the psychiatrist is an agent of society: he controls the lives of patients and relieves their relatives and society of the problems unwanted persons present. In his other role, the psychiatrist is an agent of his patient: he caters to clients and helps them cope with their problems in living. One task requires coercing the "patient"; the other task is rendered impossible by the slightest threat of coercion, much less its actual exercise.

Psychiatry's original sin is its refusal to acknowledge that the relationship between the psychiatrist and the involuntary mental patient is adversarial. In other words, the psychiatrist is a double agent, pretending to serve—impartially and "scientifically"—the interests of both parties to a conflict: the mental patient and his psychiatric opponents, such as family members, employers, and courts. This is the source of virtually all of the problems that beset mental health legislation and mental health policy. It is also why the history of psychiatry is synonymous with the history of so-called psychiatric reform, each revision further disordering the system, stimulating calls for new reforms.

Psychiatric Slavery as Protection from Dangerousness

The notion of "dangerousness to self or others" is, nominally, a medical concept, justifying—indeed, requiring—medical intervention. Yet, once a person is characterized as "dangerous to himself or others," non-psychiatric physicians typically refuse to treat him, even with his consent, while psychiatric physicians insist on treating him, even against his will.

According to a study reported in the *British Journal of Medicine*, "violent, threatening, or abusive behavior is the main reason why general practitioners remove patients from their lists."[50] No study is needed to tell us that it is precisely such behavior that characterizes the conduct of the (hospital) psychiatrists' preferred clientele; indeed, precisely such behavior is required to justify prolonged residence in a mental hospital. In plain English, regular physicians, like most people, shun associating with violent individuals. Conversely, policemen, prison guards, and psychiatrists earn their living by associating with ("caring for") violent individuals.

Overtly and nominally, psychiatrists are physicians, medical specialists; their medical identity is well recognized and not disputed. Covertly and actually, they are judges and jailers; their identity as agents of the judicial and penal systems is not well recognized and is often disputed and even denied. However, it does not require a semantic autopsy on the word "dangerous" to recognize that by so qualifying a person, we stigmatize and cast him out of society. We regularly use the adjective "dangerous" in lieu of the injunction "avoid!"— as in calling certain drugs or high tension wires "dangerous."

We use the term "dangerousness" as a medical-legal-rhetorical device to rationalize and justify certain social practices. We call persons who hallucinate or hear voices "dangerous," because we need to justify incarcerating them, but we do not call persons infected with the human immunodeficiency virus (HIV) "dangerous," because we don't want to incarcerate them. Patients with AIDS are more dangerous, and more demonstrably dangerous, to others than are patients with mental diseases. Yet, physicians have only limited power to interfere in the lives of such persons, and have no power whatever to treat them against their will.[51] In summary:

- Preventive detention is contrary to the letter and spirit of English and American law. Masked as psychiatric treatment, preventive incarceration is still preventive detention.

- It is absurd to equate dangerousness to self with dangerousness to others. Killing oneself is not a criminal offense. Killing another person is the quintessential criminal offense.

- Delegating to psychiatrists the task of forcibly protecting persons from dangerousness to self or others protects neither individuals nor the community, but opens a Pandora's box of problems.[52] Law and medicine are equally complicit in uncritically accepting the rhetoric of dangerousness as a justification for psychiatric coercion.

Conclusions

After the Civil War, social controls based on notions of race and domestic dependency began to be replaced with social controls based on ideas of illness and medical dependency, especially mental illness and the dangerousness attributed to it. The old masters needed workers coerced into submission. The new masters need patients coerced into submission. The result is the nearly worldwide, virtually unchallenged growth and popularity of pharmacratic-psychiatric social controls.[53] The essence of chattel slavery was involuntary labor, an activity forcibly imposed by master on slave.

The essence of psychiatric slavery is involuntary uselessness, a passivity forcibly imposed by psychiatric master on psychiatric slave. *Cui bono?* In a society based on black slavery and trade among free persons, the slave was useful as a degraded producer: his involuntary labor and inferior status provided material comfort, leisure, and social superiority for the slave owner, his family, and white society. In a society based on psychiatric slavery and trade among non-patients, the psychiatric slave is useful as a degraded dependent: his involuntary role as dangerous mental patient and his inferior status provide employment, existential security, and social superiority for the psychiatrist, his profession, and the mentally healthy members of society.

Few people believed or believe in equal human status for blacks and whites. In the past, the result was slavery and Jim Crow laws— "separate but equal"; today, the result is affirmative action and racial quotas. Similarly, few people believe in equal human status for mental patients and non-mental patients. The result is psychiatric slavery and psychiatric Jim Crow laws—"unequal and separate."

2

The Psychiatric Slave Status:
From Dred Scott to *Tarasoff*

Slavery was put down in America, not in consequence of any action on the part of the slaves, or even any express desire on their part that they should be free. It was put down entirely through the grossly illegal conduct of certain agitators in Boston and elsewhere, who were not slaves themselves...nor had anything to do with the question really...from the slaves themselves they received, not merely very little assistance, but hardly any sympathy, even.

—Oscar Wilde (1854-1900)[1]

Psychoanalysis is a science conducted by lunatics for lunatics. They are generally concerned with proving that people are irresponsible; and they certainly succeed in proving that some people are.

—Gilbert K. Chesterton (1874-1936)[2]

One of the most hallowed myths of American history is that Abraham Lincoln (1809-1864), often referred to as "The Great Emancipator," waged the Civil War to free the slaves. Not once did Lincoln call for the immediate emancipation of all slaves. The famously misnamed Emancipation Proclamation freed only "persons held as slaves within any State or designated part of a State, the people whereof shall then be in rebellion against the United States." The paragraph enumerating the territories affected ended with the caveat that in the areas not listed, the legal statuses of slaves "are for the present, left precisely as if this proclamation were not issued."

The claim that drugs and deinstitutionalization have freed mental patients from the shackles of mental illness and the sordidness of state mental hospitals has become a similar emancipation legend, reprising the nineteenth-century legend of Pinel's striking the chains off madmen.[3]

Lincoln did not liberate slaves, Pinel did not free mental patients, and drugs and deinstitutionalization did not end psychiatric slavery.

35

To the contrary, each of these alleged acts of liberation consisted of a new, "reformed" version of the older form of oppression, masquerading as freedom for the oppressed. Plantation slavery was replaced by Jim Crow laws, racial segregation, and pervasive discrimination based on racial stigmatization. The chains of the pre-Pinel era were replaced by the unlimited powers of a well-organized cadre of "asylum doctors," legitimized by mental health laws. State hospital-style psychiatric slavery was replaced by the Jim Crow psychiatry of outpatient commitment, forced drugging, and pervasive coercive paternalism.

From its very foundation, the United States of America was a "house divided"—half free and half slave. Many of the Founders preached liberty, but practiced slavery.[4] Were slaves property or persons? The legal argument about the status of the chattel slave came to a head in the petition for freedom of the slave, Dred Scott. His unsuccessful plea remains to this day the most famous case ever decided by the Supreme Court.

Scott v. Sanford, 60 U.S. 393, 1856.

The story of Dred Scott, and the decision named after him, has been told and retold in countless books, encyclopedias, and journal articles. I shall briefly summarize the relevant facts.[5]

Dred Scott was born in 1799, in Virginia, as a slave of the Peter Blow family. He spent his life as a slave and never learned to read or write. In 1830, the Blow family moved to St. Louis and sold Scott to Dr. John Emerson, a military surgeon stationed at Jefferson Barracks, south of St. Louis. Over the next twelve years Scott married, had two children, and accompanied Emerson to posts in Illinois and the Wisconsin Territory, where Congress prohibited slavery under the rules of the Missouri Compromise. In 1842, the Scott family returned to St. Louis with Dr. Emerson and his wife Irene. A year later, Emerson having died, the Scotts became Mrs. Emerson's property.

In 1846, supported by abolitionists, Dred Scott and his wife sued Mrs. Emerson for their freedom, claiming that, having been taken to and having resided in free states, the Scotts became free persons. The St. Louis Circuit Court ruled in favor of Mrs. Emerson but allowed the Scotts to refile their suit. In 1850, the jury, in a second trial, decided that the Scotts deserved to be free, based on their years of residence in the non-slave territories of Wisconsin and Illinois. Not wanting to lose such valuable property, Mrs. Emerson appealed the decision to the Missouri Supreme Court.

At this point, lawyers on both sides agreed that further appeals would be based on Dred's case alone, with findings applied equally to his wife. The Missouri State Supreme Court overruled the Circuit Court decision and returned Scott to slavery. Scott's lawyers then filed suit in the U.S. Federal Court in St. Louis, the defendant having become Mrs. Emerson's brother, John Sanford, who had assumed responsibility for John Emerson's estate. Again, the court ruled against Scott. In 1856, Scott and his lawyers appealed the case to the U.S. Supreme Court. In *Scott v. Sanford*, the Court ruled that Scott must remain a slave, that as a slave he is not a citizen of the United States and thus not eligible to bring suit in a federal court, and that as a slave he is personal property and thus has never been free.

These events are familiar. The opinions put forward by Chief Justice Roger Brooke Taney (1777-1864) and the two dissenting Associate Justices, Benjamin Robbins Curtis (1809-1874) and John McLean (1775-1861), are less so. I shall examine them with an eye toward the light they may throw on the controversy about the legal status of the mental patient today.

The Decision

Roger Taney, Chief Justice of the Supreme Court from 1836 until his death in 1864, wrote the majority opinion. He reasoned that the Constitution made no distinction between slaves and other types of property, and that was the end of the matter: "It has been settled by the decisions of the highest court in Missouri, that, by the laws of that State, a slave does not become entitled to his freedom, where the owner takes him to reside in a State where slavery is not permitted, and afterwards brings him back to Missouri."[6]

This conclusion rested on a selective interpretation of the law. For the purpose of electing representatives, and therefore the president via the electoral college, the Constitution identified slaves "as three-fifths of Persons."[7] Taney and his fellow concurring justices interpreted the law to preserve the legal status quo of the slave system. Like today's judge who commiserates with the mental patient for his misfortune while being the chief author of it, Taney commiserated with the Negro slave while insuring his status as property. He wrote:

It is difficult at this day to realize the state of public opinion in relation to that unfortunate race, which prevailed in the civilized and enlightened portions of the world at the time of the Declaration of Independence, and when the Constitution of the United States was framed and adopted... They had for more than a century before been regarded as beings of an inferior order, and altogether unfit to associate with the white race, either in social or political relations;...and that the negro might justly and lawfully be reduced to slavery for his benefit... This opinion was at that time fixed and universal in the civilized portion of the white race. It was regarded as an axiom in morals as well as in politics, which no one thought of disputing, or supposed to be open to dispute... No one of that race had ever migrated to the United States voluntarily; all of them had been brought here as articles of merchandise.[8]

Note the following parallels between the status of the chattel slave and the psychiatric slave. As the Negro is "reduced to slavery for his benefit," the mental patient is reduced to psychiatric coercion for his benefit: "Axiom[s] in morals as well as in politics, which no one thought of disputing, or supposed to be open to dispute [uphold the institution of slavery]." Axioms in morals as well as in politics, which no one thinks of disputing, or supposes to be open to dispute, uphold the institution of psychiatry.

The Dissenting Opinions

Benjamin Robbins Curtis was born in Watertown, Massachusetts and graduated from Harvard Law School in 1832. He was politically conservative and had no sympathy for abolitionists. As a young man, he had represented a slaveholder in *Commonwealth v. Aves* (1836), involving a slave owner who had brought a slave to Massachusetts. Curtis's support of the Fugitive Slave Law of 1850 led President Millard Fillmore to appoint him to the U.S. Supreme Court in 1851.[9] After Curtis supported the indictment of Massachusetts abolitionists who had tried to rescue a fugitive slave, many of his fellow Bostonians called him the "slave-catcher judge." Nevertheless, in 1857, Curtis wrote a vigorous, seventy-page dissent in the Dred Scott case and then resigned from the Court.

Curtis showed that, in 1787, blacks were in fact citizens in several of the states. Citing the ruling of an English judge, Curtis noted that, although in legal parlance slaves were not persons but property, "the moment the incapacity, the disqualification of slavery, was removed, they became persons, and were then either British subjects, or not British subjects, according as they were or were not born within the allegiance of the British King."[10] Significantly, Curtis called the slave status an "incapacity" and a "disqualification," that is, a social condition attached, as it were, to persons. When the disqualification is removed, the subject reverts to his natural state as a person. This is a far cry from viewing the Negro as a slave because it is his biological destiny and because the slave status is good for him. Curtis concluded:

> It has been often asserted that the Constitution was made exclusively by and for the white race. It has already been shown that in five of the thirteen original States, colored persons then possessed the elective franchise, and were among those by whom the Constitution was ordained and established. If so, it is not true, in point of fact, that the Constitution was made exclusively by the white race. And that it was made exclusively for the white race is, in my opinion, not only an assumption not warranted by anything in the Constitution, but contradicted by its opening declaration, that it was ordained and established by the people of the United States, for themselves and their posterity.[11]

Despite his anti-abolitionist convictions, Curtis was brave enough and honest enough to acknowledge the difference between a black person having dark skin, which is a fact, and his being a slave, which is a social attribution. This is precisely the distinction psychiatrists are neither brave enough nor honest enough to acknowledge. Some people feel depressed and commit suicide. Others are angry and commit murder. Those are facts. However, regarding such individuals as (mentally) ill and not responsible for their behavior is not a fact, it is a social attribution. The result is the creation of a special class of human beings—"dangerous mental patients"—and a special status appropriate to them—that of psychiatric slave. *Psychiatric slaves are persons from whose shoulders the laws of the United States have removed the rights and responsibilities attached to adults not so classified.*

Justice John McLean based his dissent on the classic antislavery view that slavery can be established only through positive law and cannot exist without it. That is, men, not God or biology, create slaves. McLean wrote: "[Sanford's] plea is this: 'That the plaintiff is a negro of African descent, his ancestors being of pure African blood, and were brought into this country, and sold as negro slaves.' But this does not show that he is not a citizen of Missouri... Several of the States have admitted persons of color to the right of suffrage, and in this view have recognized them as citizens; and this has been done in the slave as well as the free States."[12]

In addition to agreeing with Curtis that being (considered) a chattel slave was a negative status attribution or status disability, McLean emphasized that "slavery is emphatically a State institution." Indeed so. Psychiatric slavery is also a State institution. What else could each be? Only the state has legitimate power to impose such an invidious status on an individual against his will. McLean concluded with this condemnation of slavery: "This system was imposed upon our colonial settlements by the mother country... But we know as a historical fact, that James Madison, that great and good man, a leading member in the Federal [Constitutional] Convention, was solicitous to guard the language of that instrument so as not to convey the idea that there could be property in man. I prefer the lights of Madison, Hamilton, and Jay, as a means of construing the Constitution."[13]

Taney's decision illustrates the tragic predicament of the judge whose duty is to enforce an immoral law. If he is to be true to his professional obligation, then the judge must apply the law, not change it: he often must do the immoral thing. If he changes the law, he usurps the role of the legislature and the electorate. Thus, he must choose between being a good judge and being a good man. He could, of course, choose to quit his job. Similar considerations apply to modern judges called upon to implement drug laws and mental health laws.

The Psychiatrist's "Duty to Warn"

By the beginning of the twentieth century, the deleterious medical consequences of smoking were well established and well known, especially by physicians. Nevertheless, smoking was common practice among psychiatrists and psychoanalysts, notably Sigmund Freud. In the 1950s, when I was a young analyst, all of my colleagues smoked. Many died young of cardiac or pulmonary disease. It would not have occurred to them to blame their habit, which they regarded and paraded as an emblem of "psychological maturity," on cigarette manufacturers.

Suicide was also a familiar occurrence among the patients of the early psychoanalysts (as well as among the analysts). It would not have occurred to the patients' relatives to blame the subject's death on his analyst. As late as the 1960s, no one would have dreamed of suing a psychoanalyst for medical negligence because his patient killed himself or, more absurdly still, because the patient killed someone else. It did not yet occur to lawyers and judges that psychoanalysts had the duty to forcibly control their patients and that, if they failed to restrain them from "dangerousness," the psychoanalysts were guilty of malpractice. In those bygone days people still believed that there was a fundamental difference between protecting free adults from dangerous others, which was a duty the state owed the citizen, and protecting free adults from themselves, which was a duty each person owed himself. Furthermore, the idea that the psychiatrist was so omnipotent as to be able to predict a free person's behavior and had the duty to prevent him from killing himself or others was unthinkable.

All that has changed. Today, we "know" better: modern psychiatry has established, as "scientific facts," that acts injurious to oneself and/or others are due to mental-brain diseases, and that the actor who engages in such behaviors is therefore not responsible for them. Viewing such acts as the consequences of preventable and treatable diseases leads logically to blaming physicians for not preventing them. Not by coincidence, the practice of holding psychiatrists responsible for the destructive and self-destructive acts of their private psychotherapy patients is roughly concurrent with the practice of holding tobacco companies responsible for the free adult's habit of smoking cigarettes.

The more firmly the metaphor of mental illness becomes literalized, the more persuasive the following propositions become: destructive and self-destructive acts, especially by individuals with psychiatric diagnoses, are the products of mental illness; such acts are foreseeable and preventable by psychiatrists; psychiatrists are therefore responsible for the misbehavior of their patients.

These ideas have had momentous consequences for law, psychiatry, and society. Every psychiatrist and psychotherapist has been transformed into an undercover agent for the psychiatric slave system; every ostensibly *private* psychotherapeutic relationship has been moved into the sphere of *public* health medicine and "harm" prevention; every therapist who defies the reporting laws is an actual or potential defendant in an unwinnable malpractice suit. In short, the principles and practices of the psychiatric slave system have been extended from the closed ward of the mental hospital into the open world of everyday life—especially the private practice of contractual psychotherapy.

To be sure, mental health laws have always empowered psychiatrists to treat committable persons as psychiatric slaves. However, since the precedent-setting *Tarasoff* case, psychiatric reporting laws and the threat of tort litigation compel psychiatrists to treat persons considered not committable as psychiatric slaves as well: today, mental patients are either *de facto* psychiatric slaves, psychiatric slaves "on probation," or potential psychiatric slaves.

Tarasoff: *The Psychiatrist's Duty to Protect Third Parties*

Perhaps the most dramatic illustration of the expansion of psychiatric slavery is the invention of the legal-psychiatric doctrine of the psychiatrist's "duty to warn." The *McNaghten* case established insanity-as-a-disease as a valid scientific-medical element in criminal law, essential for the rationale of the insanity defense and insanity verdict.[14] Similarly, the *Tarasoff* case established the psychiatrist's duty to warn as a valid scientific-therapeutic element in civil law— essential for the rationale of the malpractice claim and jury award of damages for the psychiatrist's "failure to warn." The insanity defense clearly favors the economic and existential interests of the psychiatrist, whereas the principle of the duty to warn seemingly disfavors his interests. Actually, because both measures strengthen the bonds between law and psychiatry and legitimize psychiatric slavery, both promote the psychiatrists interests.

The basic facts of the Tarasoff case are as follows. In 1969, Prosenjit Poddar, a student at the University of California in Berkeley, formed a romantic attachment to a fellow student, Tatiana Tarasoff. She rebuffed him. He became depressed and voluntarily sought the help of a psychologist at the university health service. The psychologist became concerned that Poddar might harm Ms. Tarasoff, confided his fears to two supervising psychiatrists, planned to commit the patient, and asked the campus police to pick him up. The police did so. However, after interviewing Poddar, the officers concluded that he was rational and not dangerous, and let him go. (Policemen are not expected to make similar judgments about cancer or heart disease.)

Mr. Poddar never returned to see his "therapist." Realizing that denouncing Poddar might not have been a good idea, the psychologist panicked and decided to make no further move. Two months later, Mr. Poddar killed Ms. Tarasoff. Ms. Tarasoff's parents sued the therapist, his supervisors, and the campus police for failing to detain the patient and for failing to inform them, the parents, of the danger Poddar posed to their daughter.

The California Supreme Court ruled that the case could proceed to trial, because it is in the nature of the work of psychotherapists that they "determine, or should determine, that a patient presents a serious danger of violence to another." Accordingly, therapists have a duty to take whatever steps are necessary to protect the patient's intended victim. The source of this duty lies in the "special relationship" that exists between therapist and patient.[15] The plaintiffs' successful malpractice suit set a dramatic precedent for psychiatric practice.

The *Tarasoff* ruling is an instance of the proverbial chickens coming home to roost. Hospital psychiatrists have always had a duty to protect patients from committing suicide, and society from being harmed by patients. The legal and medical basis for these duties was that by committing dangerous mental patients, psychiatrists implicitly assert that they possess special knowledge and skills concerning the diagnosis and prediction of dangerousness. Some psychiatrists, limiting their work to the private practice of psychotherapy and psychoanalysis, rejected this premise, refused to work in state mental hospitals, and did not seek hospital privileges in private mental hospitals. The claim that psychiatrists possess special knowledge and skills concerning the diagnosis and prediction of dangerousness continues to undergird the psychiatrist's power to commit. The *Tarasoff* decision extends this classic rationale and duty from the mental hospital to any professional relationship between therapist and patient.

Interpreting the Tarasoff Decision

The organizers of the 1980 annual meeting of the American College of Forensic Psychiatry invited "king of torts" attorney Melvin M. Belli to comment on the Tarasoff case, and me to comment on Belli's paper.[16] After paying lip service to the importance of confidentiality in psychotherapy, Belli declared that the time when the law respected such confidentiality was passé: "The trend toward imposing liability on a psychotherapist for failing to inform on his dangerous patients is now firmly established. The question no longer is whether the therapist ethically may disclose such information. If the therapist unyieldingly clings to his old ethical considerations and refuses to divulge this material, the simple truth is that he will find himself having to pay a jury's verdict of $1 million or more in a wrongful death action."[17] Belli was right: he was simply reminding the audience of how things were; he was not saying how things ought to be. In my reply I observed that if the psychotherapeutic relationship is truly confidential,

there is no one to witness what transpires between therapist and client; hence there is no way for anyone to ascertain what the therapist thinks about the patient's so-called 'dangerous propensities'... Belli assumes...that it is the business of psychotherapists to predict what their clients will do. But this is absurd. The patient does not pay the therapist to have his or her behavior predicted...the issue of predicting patient behavior simply has no relevance to the private psychotherapy situation: the therapist is the patient's hired servant, not his parole officer.[18]

In the *Tarasoff* case, the therapist conducted himself as if he had been the patient's parole officer: he put in his records and informed two psychiatrists and the campus police that he believed Mr. Poddar was dangerous to Ms. Tarasoff. I concluded that if a therapist believes that his patient poses a threat to another person, the therapist's ethically proper response ought to be the same as if the patient were to pose a threat to the therapist: he ought to terminate the relationship.[19]

The relationship between Mr. Poddar and his therapist was neither private nor confidential. The therapist was a psychologist-employee of the university; he communicated his concerns about Poddar to others, including the campus police; his behavior implied that he believed that he had a duty to restrain the patient. It is likely, moreover, that denouncing Poddar to the police influenced Poddar's behavior. Being betrayed by his therapist, being apprehended by the police, and fearing psychiatric harassment and perhaps incarceration might well have contributed to Poddar's decision to kill Ms. Tarasoff. Under these circumstances, the therapist could hardly claim that he was unaware of the patient's dangerousness or that his job was to counsel, not control, the patient. Had the relationship between Mr. Poddar and his therapist been based on the classic principles of agency and confidentiality, there would have been no evidence of what Mr. Poddar told his therapist, and there might not have been a *Tarasoff* case.

Individual psychotherapy—in contrast to family therapy, group therapy, and other types of counseling—is, by definition, a private, confidential relationship between two persons: a therapist and a client or patient. Like the confessional, confidential psychotherapy allows for the presence of no third person or party. Because the therapist's participation in insurance coverage negates the privacy of the relationship, and because the law no longer protects the therapist who wants to keep his patient's communications confidential, genuine psychotherapy is now an oxymoron and an anachronism.[20]

The Duty to Rescue: Psychiatry Embraces Tarasoff

With its antennae carefully tuned to the changing political-economic climate on which it depends, organized psychiatry quickly embraced the *Tarasoff* ruling. Psychiatrists saw the ruling as a fresh opportunity to reinforce their image as the protectors of both the patient and the public and thus expand their powers. The American Psychiatric Association's new "policy for therapist confidentiality requires mental-health professionals to take actions that might violate confidentiality if a patient explicitly threatens to kill or seriously injure someone."[21] "It is disturbing," declares Paul S. Appelbaum, president of the APA and professor of psychiatry at the University of Massachusetts in Worcester, "that therapists aware of such an explicit threat to an innocent young woman [as in the Tarasoff case] should elect not to reveal it to her, while taking no other measures to reduce the risk she faced."[22]

Appelbaum embraces the duty to warn even though he recognizes that the public remains deceived about the role of the therapist as double agent: "Patients in a wide variety of jurisdictions seem remarkably unaware of the legal rules governing confidentiality in psychotherapeutic treatment. Studies have shown consistently that most persons in or out of therapy believe that their communications will be kept confidential."[23] Since the mental health misinformation flooding the media is silent regarding the risk associated with visiting a psychiatrist, this is hardly surprising.

In Appelbaum's view, entrapment is, in psychotherapy, enablement: "Therapists recognized that they could reach out to the part of their patients' personalities that resisted the idea of violence, in an attempt to form an alliance that would prevent the act from occurring...patients could be kept uninformed of this duty [to warn] until a situation arose in which it might be relevant." Translation: Keep the patient in the dark about the rules of the therapeutic game; let him think the psychiatrist will keep his communications confidential; inform him that he is about to be denounced and delivered to his enemies, in his own best interest, only after he has been entrapped and cannot escape; define such psychiatric conduct as a higher form of morality and essential for therapy.

Appelbaum concludes: "In principle, the duty to protect is difficult to reject, especially for members of a profession dedicated to assisting others in need. Indeed, I suspect that...by seeking to guard potential victims of their patients from harm, clinicians as a group would endorse the trend toward broader duties to rescue."[24] In 1988— twelve years after the *Tarasoff* case—the APA formally defined the psychiatrist's proper social role as one of double agency, declaring that "breaching confidentiality is acceptable when required to protect third parties."[25]

This is a preposterously conceited conception of the psychiatrist's role as all-purpose do-gooder. The priest hearing confessions has no duty to protect third parties from the future acts of penitents. The criminal defense lawyer has no duty to protect third parties from violence by clients. The librarian has no duty to protect third parties from harm by patrons.[26] Are priests, lawyers, and librarians less moral than psychiatrists? Or are they only less corrupt and less eager to be toadies of the state? It should be perfectly clear that the courts have appointed psychiatrists to protect not only mental patients from themselves but also third parties from mental patients—and psychiatrists have eagerly complied.

We have come a long way. In a few decades, psychiatric and legal agents of the therapeutic state managed to transform psychotherapy from a confidential relationship between a helper and a person being helped into its opposite, "a special relationship...*based on the psychiatrist's predictive powers and ability to control the patient.*"[27] Formerly, safeguarding the patient's confidences was considered a prerequisite for effective psychotherapy. Now, betraying them to authorities of the state is considered essential for legally appropriate psychotherapy. An expert on mental health law explains: "The assumptions upon which the psychotherapist-patient privilege rests have been challenged in a series of empirical studies. These 'privilege studies' suggest that the presence or absence of absolute psychotherapist-patient privilege actually has little impact upon a patient's willingness to reveal personal thoughts to a psychotherapist...*the removal of the psychotherapist-patient privilege could be therapeutically beneficial.*"[28]

This kind of reasoning depends, just as classical psychoanalytic reasoning depended, on the infinitely elastic, metaphorical use of the term "therapy." Since there is no illness in mental illness, and no therapy in psychotherapy, anything a person accredited as speaking for psychiatry and psychotherapy wants to call "illness" or "therapy" is, *ipso facto*, illness and therapy.[29] What makes the supporters of therapeutic jurisprudence recommend betraying patients to law enforcement authorities therapeutic? Their concept of the goal of psychotherapy: "The therapeutic goal of disposing of the absolute psychotherapist-patient privilege is the prevention of harmful behavior before it occurs... Prevention not only safeguards against injury to people and society as a whole, but also benefits the person whose harmful behavior has been prevented. The patient avoids incarceration, commitment, fines, and other forms of legal liability."[30] This assertion is patently false. The "potential" child molester, betrayed by the therapist, may be confined for decades, perhaps for life. The "potential" suicide, reported to the police, is often committed to a mental hospital for unwanted treatment.

Many therapists recognize that their new role has turned them into the perpetrators of gravely immoral conduct. Queried about his views regarding the duty to report "patient dangerousness," one therapist stated: "Oh, I hate it... I don't want to be a social policeman... I know I have to do it. And I agonize for hours afterwards. Then I say, 'I'm going to quit'... I never like myself after I do it."[31] Another reports: "I get angry about having to be put in this position of reporting."[32]

Aided and abetted by the law, American psychiatrists assumed the role of universal rescuer and assigned their fellow citizens to the role of persons needing to be rescued by them. Moreover, psychiatrists are not the only persons who are now expected to detect mental illness and dangerousness in their fellow human beings. Virtually every one is, especially individuals privy to personal information about people, such as beauticians, hair dressers, employers, fellow workers, teachers, and even adolescents and elementary school students. The government exhorts them all to join a patriotic army of mental health informants.[33] The result of this national mental health mobilization is a false sense of safety purchased at the cost of undermining intimate human bonds. I believe Americans will learn to regret this passion for protection from nonexistent illness and nondetectable dangerousness. (That lay persons are not expected to be able to diagnose real diseases does not seem to shake peoples' belief in the dogma that mental illness is like any other illness.)

The "Duty to Warn" and the Psychiatric Redistribution of Responsibility

The insanity defense implies that the mental patient is not responsible for his criminal act. The duty to warn doctrine implies that the psychiatrist may be held responsible for his patient's self-destructive or criminal acts. Such principles have far-reaching consequences, some intended, some not intended.

For the patient, the main consequence of the doctrine of the duty to warn is that he may find himself entrapped into the role of involuntary mental hospital inmate. For the psychiatrist, the doctrine's main consequence is that once he accepts a person as a patient, he, the therapist, is obligated to prevent his patient from engaging in self-harm, suicide, assault, and homicide. The following scenario illustrates this problem. A woman complains to her family physician that she feels depressed. The physician makes a diagnosis of depression and refers her to a psychiatrist. The psychiatrist who accepts the woman as a patient is in a bind. Like any person, this woman might kill herself. If she does, the psychiatrist is likely to be sued for malpractice by the woman's family. Hence, once the patient mentions suicide, the psychiatrist must insist that the patient admit herself to the hospital, or he must call the police and inform them that the patient is "mentally ill and dangerous to herself" and refuses "voluntary" psychiatric hospitalization.

The patient's non-responsibility and the therapist's liability do not stop there. Here is another scenario. The patient, a middle-aged woman, tells the therapist that her parents sexually abused her when she was an infant. Therapist and patient engage in a discussion of sexual abuse. The patient then publicly accuses her elderly parents of sexual abuse. The parents deny the charge and sue the therapist for making their daughter have false beliefs about them. This is not an imaginary scenario. It is the summary of several such cases.[34]

Psychotherapists form many fallacious ideas about their patients and communicate these ideas to them. This does not, and ought not, exempt patients from *responsibility for their actions*. A patient may sincerely believe that her parents had sexually abused her when she was a child. Obviously, as a criminal charge, such an accusation can be neither proved nor disproved. A grown woman has no reason to publicly accuse her parents of such a misdeed unless she wants to injure them. Why should a therapist be blamed for her verbal abuse of her parents? Because it is now believed that a woman would not make such an accusation if a therapist had not "implanted" the idea in the patient's mind. Hence, he, not the patient, is responsible for the injury to the parents.[35]

The economic liberal redistributes money, from producer to parasite. The psychiatric liberal redistributes responsibility, from patient to psychiatrist.

The Duty to Warn and Psychiatric Slavery

Chattel slavery was a business—some people producing and selling slaves, others buying and using them. The original producers and sellers were Africans, who caught other Africans and sold them to traders who brought them to the New World. The original buyers used slaves to satisfy their economic, personal, and sexual needs. Later, slaves were also created by reproduction.

As chattel slavery proved useful, it became an accepted social practice and institution, legitimized by a combination of custom, ideology, and law. The ideology rested on the belief that slavery was, as Jefferson Davis memorably put it, "a moral, social, and political blessing."[36] The legal legitimation of the system rested on denying that black slaves were full-fledged persons: the law defined them as "three fifths Persons" and made it possible to own them as if they were property. Hence the term "chattel slavery."

Similarly, as psychiatric slavery proved useful, it became an accepted social practice and institution, legitimized by a combination of custom, ideology, and law.[37] The ideology rests on the belief that psychiatric slavery—that is, the systematic incarceration and involuntary treatment of persons diagnosed as mentally ill—is a medical, moral, social, and political blessing.[38] The legal legitimation of the system rests on denying that mental patients are full-fledged persons: the law defines them as mentally ill, dangerous to themselves and others, and requiring psychiatric care, for their own benefit as well as for the benefit of the public. Their interaction with mental health professionals constitutes a "special relationship": mental health professionals have the power and obligation to protect mental patients from harming themselves or others, and the obligation to protect other persons from being harmed by mental patients.

We can now answer the question: How do psychiatrists acquire psychiatric slaves? The oldest method of psychiatric slave-catching consists of creating a special class of persons, originally called "the mad" or "insane," now called "the mentally ill" or "mentally ill and dangerous"; a special class of doctors, originally called "mad-doctors" and "alienists," now called "psychiatrists"; a special class of quasi-prisons, originally called "mad-houses" or "insane asylums," now called "mental hospitals"; and a special class of laws, called "mental health laws," that authorize psychiatrists to forcibly confine mental patients in mental hospitals. This method of catching slaves has been used for three hundred years and is still the basic tool of the slave catcher. Although the working of mental health laws is common knowledge, I offer the following hypothetical vignettes to illustrate their practical, everyday use.

- A young college student drops out of school, returns home, keeps to himself, eats sparingly, grows a beard, and states that he hears voices that tell him he is the Savior. His parents and doctor conclude that he suffers from schizophrenia and commit him to a mental hospital.

- A young woman with a two-week old infant becomes reclusive, stays in bed and neglects the baby. She refuses medical care. Her husband and the social worker he summons call an ambulance; the paramedics take her to a mental hospital.

During the waning decades of the twentieth century, a new method of slave-catching was added to the psychiatrist's repertoire: the seemingly private psychotherapy relationship. The following hypothetical scenario is an example.

- A young man, depressed by unsatisfying work and the inability to find a wife, heeds the call of mental health propaganda and makes an appointment with a psychiatrist. The doctor is sympathetic and tells the patient that successful therapy depends on his speaking his mind candidly. The patient tells the therapist about feeling angry toward his employer. Afraid that the patient might commit a violent crime, the therapist diagnoses the patient as a dangerous paranoid schizophrenic and commits him to a mental hospital.[39]

Fugitive Slave Laws and Fugitive Mental Patient Laws

Under American chattel slavery, the slave was an object that belonged to its rightful owner. If the slave escaped or was otherwise removed from the control of his master, the latter retained his right to the slave, just as he would have retained his right to an item of stolen property. This idea, as we have seen, formed the philosophical and legal basis for the Dred Scott decision.

Like all captives, slaves had a tendency to run away from slavery. The Framers anticipated this and placed in the Constitution laws regulating the status of the fugitive slave. Article IV, Section 2, Clause 3, states: "No Person held to Service or Labour in one State, under the Laws thereof, escaping into another, shall, in Consequence of any Law or Regulation therein, be discharged from such Service or Labour, but shall be delivered up on Claim of the Party to whom such Service or Labour may be due." In addition, a clause in the Northwest Ordinance of 1787 "provided for the return of slaves who had escaped to the free Northwest Territory." In 1793, Congress passed a fugitive slave law allowing owners to recover slaves merely by presenting proof of ownership before a magistrate. An order was then issued for the arrest and return of the escaped slaves, who were forbidden a jury trial and the right to give evidence in their own behalf. Finally, the Compromise of 1850 imposed heavy penalties on people who aided a slave's escape or interfered with a slave's recovery.[40]

Like slaves, patients incarcerated in mental hospitals also have a tendency to run away. Revealingly, the media refers to such patients as "escapees" and the law treats them not as if they were medical patients who left the hospital without medical permission, but as if they were fugitive slaves. Commitment is regulated by state laws. What happens to a mental patient who manages to escape and flee to another state? His legal status is regulated by the Interstate Compact on Mental Health (ICMH), a euphemism for what is, in fact, a set of fugitive mental patient laws. The ICMH authorizes each state to apprehend and forthwith forcibly return the escaped mental patient to the state from which he escaped.

Most state laws pertaining to the ICMH were enacted in the 1950s and have been updated since then. The ICMH for the State of Maine (1995)—a typical example of these regulations—describes the Compact's purpose as follows:

> The party states find that the proper and expeditious treatment of the mentally ill and mentally deficient can be facilitated by cooperative action, to the benefit of the patients, their families and society as a whole. The party states find that the necessity of and desirability for furnishing such care and treatment bears no primary relation to the residence or citizenship of the patient...it is the purpose of this compact and of the party states to provide the necessary legal basis for the institutionalization or other appropriate care and treatment of the mentally ill and mentally deficient under a system that recognizes the paramount importance of patient welfare and to establish the responsibilities of the party states in terms of such welfare.[41]

By entering into the ICMH, the parties agree to apprehend and return all escaped mental patients to their rightful "owners": the "state [to which the patient has escaped] shall promptly notify all appropriate authorities within and without the jurisdiction of the escape in a manner reasonably calculated to facilitate the speedy apprehension of the escapee. Immediately upon the apprehension and identification of any such dangerous or potentially dangerous patient, he shall be detained in the state where found pending disposition in accordance with law."[42]

By definition, all committed mental patients need to be hospitalized involuntarily. Fugitive mental patient laws thus apply to all such patients, and, potentially, to all voluntarily hospitalized mental patients as well.[43] Consider the following definitions of key terms in the Maine law: "'Mental illness' means mental disease to such extent that a person so afflicted requires care and treatment for his own welfare or the welfare of others or of the community... 'Patient' means any person subject to or eligible, as determined by the laws of the sending state, for institutionalization or other care, treatment or supervision pursuant to this compact."

The practical importance of the ICMH cannot be exaggerated. The following excerpt from a court's decision concerning the extradition of an escaped mental patient is illustrative. Committed to a mental hospital in Nebraska, Michael S. White fled to West Virginia, was apprehended, and sought a *habeas corpus* hearing regarding his transfer to, and *de facto* re-imprisonment in, Nebraska. In 1996, the Supreme Court of Appeals of West Virginia ruled that "One who is suffering from a debilitating mental illness and in need of treatment is neither wholly at liberty nor free of stigma."[44] This is boilerplated psychiatric jargon. White could not have been very "debilitated" if he was able to escape from a closed mental institution, make his way to another state many miles away, and sue for his freedom. But debility and mental illness had nothing to do with the matter. The real issue was dangerousness: "Clearly, there is a compelling public policy to quickly detain a dangerous or potentially dangerous patient... Thus, only a minimal amount of due process need be given...appellant was appointed counsel to represent him at a *habeas corpus* proceeding in which it was determined that he was indeed the person who escaped from the mental health facility in Nebraska."[45]

Ironically, fugitive mental patient laws are more hypocritical than were fugitive slave laws. The Supreme Court did not claim it was returning Dred Scott to his owner to benefit Scott. The framers of laws pledging support for the Interstate Compact on Mental Health make precisely that claim: they are returning the escaped mental patient to psychiatric slavery in his own best interest.

The irony is deepened by the fact that escaped slaves sometimes voluntarily returned to slavery, but I have never heard of a case of an escaped mental patient voluntarily returning to the hospital from which he escaped. In 1841, John Clemens, the father of Samuel Clemens/Mark Twain, sat on a Marion County, Missouri jury, where the accused were "three abolitionists who ushered a handful of slaves north to freedom. The slaves had returned on their own and turned in their liberators."[46]

This discussion of fugitive slaves and fugitive mental patients would be incomplete without mentioning the early medicalization of the slave's craving for freedom, that is, the discovery, in 1851, of two "diseases peculiar to negroes"—drapetomania and dysaesthesia Aethiopis. Drapetomania was defined as "the disease causing slaves to run away," while dysaesthesia Aethiopis was said to be a "hebetude of mind peculiar to negroes."[47]

This is not all. Anticipating psychiatric abuses by a century, abolitionism itself was sometimes dismissed as madness, and the most famous American abolitionist had to reject the imposition of an insanity defense. John Brown's "attorneys tried to prevent his being sentenced to the gallows by entering a plea of insanity but Brown was incensed at the idea, and announced he was as sane as they were." Frederick Douglass aptly offered this eulogy for Brown: "Mine was as the taper light; his was as the burning sun. I could live for the slave; John Brown could die for him."[48]

These early attempts to demean the Negro slave's and the white abolitionist's passion for liberty as symptoms of mental illness foreshadowed the frightening similarities between the dying system of chattel slavery and the developing system of psychiatric slavery.

Conclusions

In its pristine form, psychoanalysis—which forms the template for virtually all modern psychotherapies—was based on a contract: the patient promised to speak freely, and the analyst promised to keep the information he received confidential. When I began to practice psychoanalysis in the late 1940s, the analyst's duty to keep his patient's communications confidential was regarded as every bit as sacrosanct as the priest's in the confessional. Indeed, strict confidentiality was the very essence of true psychoanalysis. When this confidentiality began to be systematically compromised—by child analysis and training analysis—psychoanalysis ceased to exist, except in name.[49] There is good reason for this, and it is important that we understand it.

Like the confessional, psychoanalysis rests on an interpersonal situation in which one person is expected to incriminate himself, and the other person is expected to help the self-incriminating person conduct his life better. The priest offers absolution. The therapist offers understanding, explanation, and advice. As long experience with the confessional has shown, this kind of situation engenders excessive self-accusation in one party, and excessive forgiveness in the other. Penitents may feel encouraged to confess to many minor moral infractions, real and imaginary, in an effort to demonstrate the purity of their soul, a behavior called "scrupulosity." Similarly, patients in psychotherapy may feel encouraged to imagine and relate all kinds of aggressive and lurid fantasies.

If the therapist is obligated to report patients who relate fantasies of harming others, psychotherapy is transformed from a helping situation into a sting operation: instead of caring for voluntary patients, the private psychotherapist is enlisted in the army of psychiatric slave-catchers, creating involuntary patient-slaves for the psychiatric plantations. Of course, nothing remotely resembling "psychotherapy" can be practiced in such a legal-psychiatric climate.

The confidentiality of the psychotherapist-patient relationship was destroyed decades ago, largely by the insertion of third-party insurance coverage for the mythical treatment called "psychotherapy."[50] Nevertheless, the false claim that the relationship between the psychotherapist and his patient is confidential continues to be foisted on the public. The APA proudly sponsors an obscene "Mental Health Bill of Rights," guaranteeing mental patients the right to "competent and quality care...[and] *confidentiality*."[51]

The doctrine of the duty to warn brings us full circle, back to the classic concept of the mental patient as a madman, that is, an angry and violent person. The psychiatrist's duty to warn rides piggy-back on the mental patient's potentiality to harm himself or others.

3

Psychiatric Slavery as Public Health: Infection and Insanity

> Absolute government must be either despotic or paternal... If you appeal to force, you cannot also appeal to conscience.
> —*Lord Acton (1834-1902)[1]*

> Neither psychiatrists nor anyone else [have] reliably demonstrated an ability to predict future violence or "dangerousness."
> —*American Psychiatric Association (1974)[2]*

The single most important political question is: Which acts concern the actor only and hence fall outside the scope of legislative control, and which concern the public as well and hence are appropriately controlled by the state? John Stuart Mill suggested the terms "self-regarding acts" for the former class of behaviors, and "other-regarding acts" for the latter. Although the border between these two classes of actions is often unclear and contested, the distinction is one of the guiding principles of the free society.

Self-regarding acts range from reading books and practicing religion—rights guaranteed by the First Amendment—to engaging in certain behaviors that are actually or potentially self-destructive. Other-regarding acts range from creating a public disturbance to crimes such as driving while intoxicated, assault, and murder.

Since the latter half of the nineteenth century, socialist politics and a collectivist public health ideology have struggled to erase the boundaries between self and society, between injuring oneself and injuring others. "Every injury to the health of the individual is, so far as it goes, a public injury," declared English philosopher Thomas Hill Green (1836-1882).[3] With this dictum as their creed, health statists—led by psychiatrists—have largely succeeded in convincing Americans that such radically different behaviors as injuring or killing oneself and injuring or killing others are similar and, indeed, belong in the same moral class. The result is a fudging of the differences between dangerousness to self and dangerousness to others, and a blurring of the separation between the private sphere, free of state regulation, and the public sphere, the object of state regulation.

The principal political objection to the key psychiatric term "dangerousness to self and others" is that it combines—in a single, scientific-sounding formula—two radically different kinds of dangerousness. One is taking risks with one's own body and life, the *sine qua non* of what we mean by individual liberty. The other is deliberately endangering or injuring the bodies and lives of others, acts that epitomize criminal offenses. Furthermore, the psychiatric formula of "dangerousness to self and others" is highly susceptible to changing medical, political, and social fashions. Prior to 1973, homosexuality constituted such dangerousness; since then it does not. Today, it is the private use of heroin that counts as dangerousness, and its public control by the court-mandated use of methadone that qualifies as treatment. At the same time, engaging in unsafe sexual practices and a wide range of risky behaviors categorized as sports are not included in the sphere of public dangerousness.

Erroneously perceived as a proclivity belonging to a person, the phrase "dangerousness to self and others" functions as an incantation, a rhetorical device justifying the abolition of the distinction between self-regarding and other-regarding behaviors. The result is that any self-regarding conduct, considered at the moment socially repugnant, may be defined as other-regarding, hence justifying its control by the state. *The legal-psychiatric use of the doctrine of "dangerousness to self and others" represents the most radical, yet least recognized, attack on the principle of separating the private sphere from the public sphere.* Seemingly, the phrase names a condition or predisposition. In practice, it is typically attributed to a person with a psychiatric diagnosis, to justify depriving him of liberty, and rationalize the deprivation of liberty as therapy for illness, not punishment for crime.

Psychiatry as a Branch of Public Health Medicine

Modern psychiatry rests on the false premise that mental illnesses are brain diseases treatable with drugs. Political correctness requires that we accept this premise and the practices it entails as the products of modern neuroscience and the procedures of humane social control. As science, this is bunk, because it confuses personal conduct with biological condition. As social control, it is despotism, subjecting innocent individuals to incarceration. The following vignette illustrates the actual working of the system.

On the morning of December 20, 2000, Cathy Cartwright set fire to her apartment and then walked to McDonald's for breakfast. Her husband and one of her daughters were asleep. The apartment complex, housing 11 families, burned to the ground. Miraculously, all the occupants escaped. Property damage was estimated at $1.5 million. Many of the residents had no insurance. Who was Cathy Cartwright?

> Cathy Cartwright, 39, threw rocks at cars on I-275, set her house in Detroit on fire three times without being criminally charged and threatened to kill herself and her family members on several occasions... "If you leave me out here, I will hurt someone," Cartwright warned Detroit police outside her burning home in 1991... June 1993: John Cartwright said his wife was threatening to hurt everyone. October 1995: A Detroit police officer said Cathy Cartwright said she wanted to kill herself and asked the officer to shoot her. January 1996: A Detroit police officer responded to a call about Cartwright with a gun threatening to shoot somebody in the area. June 1996: ...John Cartwright said his wife...constantly asked him and his daughters to kill her.[4]

Cartwright made it clear that she did not want to be a responsible wife and mother, that she could not bear the burden of living and had not the courage to kill herself—in short, she wanted others to take care of her or kill her. But no one listened. Instead, she was incarcerated in a mental hospital, medicated, and discharged with a prescription for drugs she had no intention to take. When we listen through psychiatry-filtered ears, we can no longer hear, much less understand, what the Cathy Cartwrights of the world tell us.

The Nature and Scope of Public Health Medicine

The *Oxford Textbook of Public Health* defines public health as "the process of mobilizing local, state, national, and international resources to solve the major health problems affecting communities."[5] By definition, public health is concerned with the health of the public, not the health of the private person. Accordingly, the scope of public health laws must be limited to protecting the public. Extending their scope to encompass "protecting" private persons destroys privacy and liberty.

In free societies, agriculture, manufacturing, trade, religion, and health care—providing material, spiritual, and medical goods and services to individuals—are considered to belong in the private sphere. These functions are performed consensually, by agreement between free persons. No one can be compelled to farm, manufacture, worship, or receive medical or surgical treatment against his will.

In contrast, the criminal justice system, public health system, and psychiatry—protecting the public from lawlessness, certain contagious diseases and toxins, and dangerous mental patients—are considered to belong in the public sphere. These functions are performed coercively, by agents of the state imposing their "services" on individuals, for the benefit of the community. People can be compelled by force to obey criminal laws, public health laws, and mental health laws. The scope of individual liberty thus depends not only on what we consider to be a crime or a dangerous disease, but also on whom we consider to be dangerous.

Controlling voluntary self-destructive acts used to be considered one's own business, called prudence and self-control. Controlling voluntary acts injurious to others used to be the business of legislators, prosecutors, judges, juries, and prison wardens, and was called punishment and deterrence. The doctor's business used to be to diagnose and treat disease, with the consent of the patient. Now, politicians define disease, and doctors control bad behavior. Active children, violent adolescents, anxious adults, sad seniors, and anomic assassins are believed to act as they do because of the diseases that are presumed to afflict them.

Psychiatry and public health exhibit two obvious similarities. Both are concerned with protecting the public from ill health, and both expend much effort on expanding the scope and power of their respective domains. Mental health and public health professionals lead the armies of medicalization toward their shared goal of controlling all human behavior by pharmacratic regulations.[6]

As problems considered "health problems" expand, so does the scope of public health medicine. Traditionally, the public health physician was concerned with issues such as sewage disposal, the provision of potable water, and the spread of certain infectious diseases, such as cholera, tuberculosis, typhoid fever, and venereal diseases. His modern counterpart is concerned with "lifestyle diseases" that stem from an overly rich diet, the use of alcohol, cigarettes, illegal drugs, and violence against oneself and others. Like psychiatrists,

public health physicians now offer excuses for a person's misbehavior, blaming his conduct not on bad choices but on abstractions
such as "social conditions" or on third parties with deep pockets,
exemplified by tobacco companies.

Blaming murder and suicide on guns, and smoking on tobacco
companies, has become the hallmark of the modern, liberal-scien-
tific physician. In 1992, then Surgeon General C. Everett Koop and
then Editor-in-Chief of the *Journal of the American Medical Association* (*JAMA*) George D. Lundberg declared: "One million U.S.
inhabitants die prematurely each year as a result of intentional homicide or suicide... We believe violence in America to be a public
health emergency."[7] Articles about smoking, violence, and war are
staples in the pages of the *JAMA*.[8] According to Jeremiah Barondess,
president of the New York Academy of Medicine, the average doctor's
examination should "include questions not only about a patient's
consumption of red meat and alcohol, but of ammunition, too."[9]

This thinking confuses the causes of disease with disease. The
tubercle bacillus is a microbe, not a disease; if inhaled, it causes
tuberculosis. Disease is something that happens to the subject, typically against his will. A sleeping person cannot shoot himself or
commit a crime, but he can acquire a disease, for example, become
infected with malaria.[10] Shooting a person is an act, the choice and
deed of a moral agent.

The person with a gun and the person with infectious tuberculosis
pose very different kinds of dangers. The former does not, passively,
give off bullets or bullet wounds; to be a danger, he must aim the
gun at someone and fire it, i.e. engage in a voluntary act. Being in
the same room or on the same airplane with a person who has a gun
does not, *per se*, constitute a danger to others. On the contrary, under certain circumstances, it is precisely the possession of a gun that
protects people from dangerous persons. In contrast, the breath of
the person with infectious tuberculosis gives off tubercle bacilli. Such
a person is dangerous to others who occupy the same air space as he
does by his mere presence. Neither the infected person nor the person at risk needs to engage in any other action.

In the case of many illnesses now considered public health problems, the potential victim is safe from harm unless he deliberately
engages in certain behaviors, such as smoking, drinking too much,
overeating, engaging in dangerous sexual behavior, and so forth.
The celibate person is not endangered by the patient with infectious

venereal diseases. The person with temperate habits is not at risk of developing alcoholism or obesity.[11]

The aim of public health is singular: preventing healthy persons from getting ill. The prototypical act of legal coercion justified on the ground of protecting the public from illness is quarantining infectious animals and persons. Treating sick persons is a public health concern only as a means of preventing the spread of disease. In contrast, the aims of psychiatry are dual: preventing dangerousness to self and others, and promising treatment for mental illness. Indeed, delivering treatment to the mental patient that, because of his illness, the patient rejects, is now a major justification for psychiatric coercion, both in and outside the mental hospital.

Public Psychiatry

Psychiatrists define public psychiatry as the care of severely ill mental patients. Actually, the term is a euphemism for involuntary psychiatry: public psychiatry is public health control masquerading as private health care.

Chattel slavery rested on the denial that the Negro was a person. Psychiatric slavery rests on the denial that the person with a psychiatric diagnosis is a person with the ability and right to make decisions about his own life. To this, the doctrine of psychiatric slavery adds the lie that psychiatric imprisonment is hospitalization. The result is that psychiatrists systematically misdefine public psychiatry and misdescribe its true aim. The advertisement for a "Public Psychiatry Fellowship" at Columbia University College of Physicians and Surgeons is typical. It states: "'Public' Psychiatry refers to the use of clinical techniques, management skills and evaluation strategies within established institutions *serving populations with social as well as psychiatric needs*: patients with severe mental illness and other major social psychiatric problems such as substance abuse, homelessness and AIDS, as well as members of poor urban and suburban minorities."[12] Not a word is said about social control.

The primary aim of the practicing non-psychiatric physician is to diagnose and treat his patient's illness and, more generally, relieve his distress. Such a physician, too, has certain obligations to the state, for example, to report certain diseases; but this duty plays a very small role, or often no role at all, in his practice. The point is that, in medicine, the roles of private practitioner and public health physician are distinct and separate, whereas in psychiatry, they are not.

Psychiatrists are obligated to play both roles at all times. Moreover, prominent psychiatrists have always insisted that public psychiatry constitutes the core of the profession, and tended to disdain private psychiatry as a frill.[13] This is still the case. William Edwin Fann, professor of psychiatry at Baylor University in Houston, remarks: "Our medical specialty needs a clearer definition of itself. Most of us who have spent our *careers in public psychiatry* would likely insist that training be directed toward *care of the most severely ill*."[14]

Supporters of psychiatric slavery always justified their use of force by defining it as protection of the best interests of both the patient and the public. To this, they have now added protecting the mental patient's civil rights as well. Camus spoke bitterly of "the day when crime dons the apparel of innocence." Today, the foe of human rights dons the apparel of the friend of human rights. Public health physicians and psychiatrists proclaim: "The means to provide the mentally ill with the rights taken for granted by the vast majority of people in industrialized nations are now becoming available. Assuring these rights to those suffering from mental illness must become part of the public health agenda."[15] Why do mental patients need physicians to "provide" them with rights? Because it was psychiatric physicians who robbed them of their rights. Like arsonist-firemen who return to the scene of their crime to put out the fires they set, psychiatrists return to the scene of their crime to provide rights for the persons whose rights they have deliberately violated.

Controlling Tuberculosis and Controlling Schizophrenia

Under pressure to justify coercing schizophrenics, psychiatrists have turned to comparing schizophrenia controls with tuberculosis controls. It is an absurd comparison: *The person with tuberculosis gives others tuberculosis. The person with schizophrenia does not give others schizophrenia.* The comparison of tuberculosis with schizophrenia highlights the following points:

- Pulmonary tuberculosis is an objectively identifiable illness. With appropriate laboratory methods, it can be proved that the patient is or is not ill or contagious.

- Neither dangerousness nor schizophrenia is an objectively identifiable illness. There are no laboratory methods to measure mental illness or dangerousness. Of course, a person called "schizophrenic" can assault, rob, and kill others, just as can a person not called "schizophrenic."

- Insanity is not contagious. Under the guise of combating dangerous diseases, mental health laws attempt to purge society of persons whom psychiatrists label "dangerous."

In the English and American legal system, the state must prove that an accused is guilty; without proof of guilt, the accused cannot be punished. The person erroneously suspected of having infectious tuberculosis can be proven to be non-contagious. However, the person erroneously accused of having schizophrenia and being dangerous cannot be proven healthy or safe. More than anything else, this is what makes deprivation of liberty on psychiatric grounds incompatible with the principles of a free society.[16]

Richard Coker, a British public health physician who studied the control of tuberculosis in both the United Kingdom and the United States, states unequivocally: "*Detention* of patients with tuberculosis should be dependent on the threat they pose to *public health* and on this concept alone."[17] With respect to the treatment of the disease, "the patient's task is voluntary."[18] In other words, treatment of the disease for the benefit of the patient does not justify his coercion. This is not true for the control of mental illness. Coker acknowledges: "Since 1979 several states have changed their laws to permit involuntary commitment of mentally ill individuals *in need of treatment who are not necessarily dangerous even to themselves.*"[19]

Public health physicians in the United Kingdom emphasize that *tuberculosis control laws do not permit compulsory treatment.* "Section 37 of the United Kingdom's Public Health (Control of Disease) Act contains *no power for compulsory treatment of [tuberculosis] patients...* [It] allows only for removal to hospital and neither here nor elsewhere in current public health law is there any provision for compulsory treatment of patients. We would not like our clinical colleagues to be under the impression that the legal power to force patients to accept treatment exists."[20]

In the United States, the use of coercion to control communicable diseases is limited by similar constraints. In the 1990s, an upsurge of tuberculosis in New York City, especially among homeless AIDS patients, led to the Commissioner of Health's being authorized to issue "orders compelling a person to be examined for tuberculosis, to complete treatment, to receive treatment under direct observation, or to be detained for treatment [if he is infectious]."[21] The phrase, "treatment under direct observation"—also called "directly observed therapy" (DOT)—refers to social workers or other health care personnel visiting patients wherever they live and ascertaining that they take the prescribed medications. The workers are authorized to encourage patient compliance with *rewards,* such as food supplements, fast-food vouchers, movie passes, clothing, and money, but *cannot impose penalties for non-compliance.*

"Why," asks Coker, "has the detention of noncompliant tuberculosis patients in the 1990s not followed the model of the commitment for the mentally ill in the 1970s?"[22] Because the goal of tuberculosis control has been to minimize recourse to coercion by limiting the state's power to protecting the public from the contagious patient, eschewing the use of force to protect the patient from himself. Coker repeatedly emphasizes the limited scope of medical coercion in tuberculosis control. He writes: "In the case of any individuals with tuberculosis, it should be shown by a factual finding that he or she presents *a significant risk of harm to others...* [A] speculative risk should not justify the imposition of these public health measures... Coercion, as a tool in the public health armamentarium...should be used sparingly...and *only where a significant threat to the public health is posed."*[23] Even more emphatically, an editorial in the *New England Journal of Medicine* declares: "On the locked ward in the New York City program, [tuberculosis] patients have to agree to take their medications. *No program should have the power to force pills physically down a patient's throat."*[24]

In the case of mental health laws, the opposite principle prevails: forcing drugs down a patient's throat, or injecting them into his buttocks, is exalted as a sacred therapeutic duty. In September 2000, the Ohio Supreme Court ruled that "involuntarily committed psychiatric patients can be forced to take antipsychotic drugs *even if they are not a danger to themselves or others."*[25] What justifies their forced drugging? That "taking medication is in the patient's best interests."[26]

Mental illness, a non-disease, is the only "disease" that justifies the use of coercion *in the best interest of the coerced person.* This policy is widely praised as humane treatment based on medical science. Despite the evidence presented above, E. Fuller Torrey claims that public health laws controlling patients with tuberculosis support the forcible *treatment* of patients with schizophrenia: "Their tuberculosis could be *treated,* but not their schizophrenia. Is there something inherently different in brains and lungs? Or is it that our brains are not thinking clearly?"[27]

Psychiatry's clarion call for treatment with "medications" has been generally well received by the American public. Many people like to take drugs and like to be dominated by authorities they regard as benevolent. Carrie Fisher, writer and actress identified as "one of manic-depression's best-known champions," explains: "Bipolar disorder can be a great teacher... I feel that the medication that I'm on can handle it."[28] Valerie Fox, who identifies herself as a woman who has "suffered from schizophrenia for the past 30 years," writes: "I have been monitored for most of my adult life, and am grateful for it.. [I]f a person is living in a state of fantasy and imagination (voices and hallucinations) and is lacking free will, I believe he or she should have to receive treatment."[29]

However, neither such endorsements nor references to contagious disease control laws justify mental health laws mandating treatment of the patient. Persons with active venereal diseases are more dangerous to others, and are more demonstrably dangerous, than are persons with psychiatric diagnoses. Nevertheless, they are free to infect anyone willing to engage in a sexual act with them, and physicians have no powers to confine them, let alone forcibly treat them. (Forcible treatment of patients forms no part of the laws requiring physicians to report certain diseases, such as gonorrhea, pertussis, and salmonellosis.[30])

We confuse and mislead ourselves if we look to the principles and practices used to protect people from the dangers of infectious diseases as a model for understanding or formulating policies for protecting people from the dangers of mental diseases. We are tempted to try to control mental diseases on the model of controlling infectious diseases largely because they were the first diseases understood and conquered by scientific medicine. The response of the immune system to the pathogenic microorganism is readily analogized to a nation resisting an invading army. Thus, the war metaphor is used when we speak about microbes "attacking" the body, antibiotics as magic "bullets," doctors as "fighting" against diseases, and so forth; we use military metaphors to convey the idea that the doctor is like the soldier who protects the homeland from foreign invaders. However, people are not microbes. Thus, when we speak about the war on mental illness, we use a military metaphor to convey the idea that the state is like a doctor when it uses physicians as soldiers to protect people from themselves or to protect the public from people who might break the law. In one case, we speak about doctors helping patients to overcome diseases; in the other, about doctors preventing citizens from doing what they want to do or engaging in law-enforcement under the guise of medicine.

Modern medical wars on disease and drugs bear an uncomfortable resemblance to medieval religious wars on heretics and witches.[31] In each case, the war is waged to protect the people, but the result is their persecution and destruction. Clearly, the state is an instrument of violence, while the church is, or ought to be, an instrument of non-violence. Nevertheless, it took centuries of terrible religious wars before people began to recognize that church and state ought to get a divorce or at least a legal separation. This principle lies at the core of the founding of the United States. Yet, American states now lead the charge in refusing to view the relationship between medicine and the state the same way as they view the relationship between church and state. One reason for this may be that the physical ill health of the individual, unlike his spiritual ill health, can *directly* affect the physical health of the group. This cause and effect connection has justified certain public health measures as legitimate instruments of state coercion. Still, such reasoning cannot justify the coercive protection of *private health.* The coercive apparatus of the state ought to be as separate from the treatment of medical ill health as it is from the treatment of spiritual ill health.

The comparison of the control of mental illness with the control of infectious disease does not strengthen the case for psychiatric coercions, as psychiatrists claim. It weakens it. How much it weakens it is illustrated by a comparison of the control and decontrol of leprosy with the escalating controls of mental illness.

The Leper Colony: The Prototype of Medical Exclusion

Leprosy is one of the oldest known diseases, and the coercive segregation of lepers is the oldest example of the systematic exclusion of individuals from society on medical grounds. Since the disease was incurable, the exclusion was intended to benefit the healthy members of the community, not the patients. After World War II, antileprosy drugs rendered the segregation of leprosy patients unnecessary. A comparison of the fate of deinstitutionalized leprosy patients and deinstitutionalized mental patients further unmasks the stubborn inhumanity of psychiatrists. Regardless of whether they imprison individuals *en masse* in mental hospitals, or evict them *en masse* from them, psychiatrists reject letting patients have a voice in shaping their own fate.

A Brief History of Leprosy

Leprosy is a systemic disease caused by Mycobacterium leprae, an organism morphologically similar to the tubercle bacillus. The microorganism was discovered in 1879 by Gerhard Henrik Armauer Hansen (1841-1912), a Norwegian physician, and the illness is also known as "Hansen's disease."[32]

Long recognized as a contagious disease, the systematic segregation of leprosy patients began in the early Middle Ages. Soon, thousands of leprosaria dotted the map of Europe. Referred to as "the living death," the victims of leprosy were often treated as though they were dead; sometimes, funeral services were conducted for them, "to declare their 'death' to society."[33]

Until the 1950s, Americans who contracted leprosy were confined involuntarily at the National Leprosarium in Carville, Louisiana. The leprosarium opened in 1894, and closed in June 1999. Originally a sugar plantation, the facility, in the 1940s, was renamed the Gillis W. Long Hansen's Disease Center and evolved into a hospital and research center. At its height, it was home to about 600 patients and "had a band, a baseball team...a press...churches...a power plant, [and] a dairy farm."[34]

In 1935, it was discovered that the sulfa and sulfone drugs developed by Gerhardt Domagk, a German chemist working for I. G. Farben, were effective against leprosy and rendered the patients non-contagious. In 1941, Guy Faget, an American physician working at the leprosarium in Carville, showed that a sulfone drug, promin, was effective against leprosy. Soon, other anti-leprosy drugs were developed. Today, a combination of three drugs—dapsone, rifampin, and clofazimine—are used to render patients non-contagious. The therapeutic control of leprosy with drugs rendered the social control of lepers legally and medically unjustified and practically unnecessary.

Deinstitutionalizing Leprosy Patients and Deinstitutionalizing Mental Patients

To the credit of the medical profession and the government, institutionalized leprosy patients no longer needing hospitalization were dealt with humanely and rationally. They were given genuine free-dom, that is, a choice over their fate crippled by long isolation from society: "The government offered patients three alternatives. They could live on their own and receive a tax-free annual stipend of $33,000 in addition to free health care and Social Security. They could be placed in a federal nursing home in nearby Baton Rouge, where most of Carville's medical staff will be relocating. Or they could stay at Carville, sectioned off in a small section of the re-vamped facility."[35]

Many patients chose to stay, which surprised some naive observ-ers. "I think the interesting part is," said one, "when the quarantine was lifted, and the people were free to go, many of them stayed...this is one of the really amazing things about Carville."[36] The leprosa-rium was indeed a prison, to start with, but, like the mental hospital, it soon became the only home the inmates had. "'I didn't ask to come here,' says Johnny Harmon, an 87-year-old retired photogra-pher who entered Carville in 1935. 'But this became my home'... Many have lived here for decades and have found a makeshift fam-ily among fellow patients and the staff. 'The worst part of the dis-ease is the stigma. People see leprosy in a movie. And that is all they know when they meet you. Here we have a safe haven.'"[37]

The similarities between the segregation of leprosy patients and mental patients are striking. What is even more striking is the con-trast between the choices that were offered deinstitutionalized lep-rosy patients and the choices that were denied deinstitutionalized mental patients. Leprosy patients were given true freedom. They could come and go as they pleased and were not forced to take antileprosy drugs. Mental patients were kept under indefinite psy-chiatric surveillance and forced to take antipsychotic drugs. The clo-sure of leprosy hospitals was accompanied by an offer of custodial care for former inmates, but the closure of state hospitals was not accompanied by such an offer. The acclaimed therapeutic control of schizophrenia with drugs did not render the social control of schizophrenics with coercive segregation legally unjustified and prac-tically unnecessary. Again, the difference is due to the fact that schizo-phrenia is not a disease but the name that we give individuals who do bad things to themselves or others.

Claims to the contrary notwithstanding, mental illnesses are *not* like other illnesses, and the dangers to the public posed by patients with mental diseases are *not* like the dangers posed by patients with communicable diseases. The terms "mental illness" and "dangerousness" have special justificatory functions in mental health laws, which are *exceptional laws*: they authorize both the preventive detention of innocent persons and the continued detention of criminals who have completed their prison sentences. Psychiatric physicians are *exceptional doctors*: they are authorized to function as both the patient's protector and his persecutor; and psychiatric institutions are *exceptional hospitals*: they are authorized to function as both hospitals and prisons.[38]

Escape from Conflict

In 1854, John C. Bucknill, M.D (1817-1897), superintendent of the asylum in Devon, England, wrote: "There is but little analogy and much contrast between the asylum and the general hospital... The comparison of the asylum to the general hospital as an argument, was fit only *ad captandum vulgus* [in order to win over the masses]."[39] This is even more true today than it was one hundred and fifty years ago. Virtually all the problems associated with the relationship between so-called severely ill mental patients and the mental health professionals who ostensibly treat them have their origin in the socially validated claim that the relationship between involuntary mental patient and psychiatrist resembles the relationship between voluntary patient and physician, rather than the relationship between slave and master. As a result, it is virtually impossible to address this root problem of psychiatry: the very act of identifying it, in terms such as I have used, is taboo. If a person diagnosed as a mental patient breaks the taboo, insisting that his relationship to "his doctor" is an adversarial one, he is dismissed as paranoid. And if a person qualified as a psychiatrist breaks this taboo, he is cast out of the profession and loses his credibility, especially as a witness in court proceedings concerning civil commitment and personal responsibility for crime.[40]

To overcome this impasse, I proposed, many years ago (in 1966), that we formally distinguish between the psychiatrist's two mutually incompatible roles: "defense psychiatrist," helping the voluntary patient pursue his own interest, and "prosecuting psychiatrist," harming the involuntary "patient" in the interest of his *de facto* adversaries.[41] Acknowledging the distinction would compel psychiatrists, patients, lawyers, and the public to recognize that problems of psychiatric coercion are matters of *conflict and power (ethics, politics)*, not matters of *disease and treatment (medicine, science)*. While the separation of these roles would offer better protection for the self-defined interests of both parties than are offered by present policies, it would destroy the tactical uses of psychiatric testimony in court. Such a proposal could become acceptable only after psychiatric slavery is abolished.

Coercive Psychiatry and the Denial of Conflict

To resolve the conflicts between the psychiatrist's duty to protect society from the dangers mental patients pose or are believed to pose, and his duty to help persons cope with the vicissitudes of life, we must not only transcend the limitations imposed on us by the established vocabulary of the mental health professions, we must also repudiate the legitimacy of psychiatric slavery.[42] The difficulties we face go far beyond psychiatry's defense of its good name and traditional privileges. The basic problem is that the public is happy to conflate and confuse the psychiatrist's mutually incompatible roles into one of healing. The following example is typical.

> *The Independent,* April 23, 2000: Janet Cresswell, the award-winning playwright who has spent the past 22 years in Broadmoor has been placed on a regime of mind-altering drugs for daring to oppose the hospital authorities... Ms Cresswell, 67, is in Broadmoor because she slashed her psychiatrist's buttocks with a vegetable knife. Yet she has been kept behind bars for 22 years. This is because she insists she is not mad and has always refused to go under the supervision of a Home Office psychiatrist... Broadmoor Hospital said last night that it was unable to comment on individual patients but... "There is an ability for a patient to be compulsorily medicated if there is a need to do so but no one can be medicated against their will without the protection of the Mental Health Act."[43]

If the interests of the patient and the psychiatrist mesh, then, like any buyer and seller, they contract and cooperate. However, if their interests conflict, then nothing short of repealing mental health laws can protect innocent individuals from becoming the victims of psychiatric violence, justified as treatment for mental illness; and nothing short of holding persons legally accountable for their behavior, regardless of their having an alleged mental illness, can protect the public from being victimized by "mental patients" whose criminal acts are attributed to mental illness.

The very terms "psychiatrist," "psychologist," "clinician," and "therapist" imply that the mental health professional's legal, moral, and professional duty entails protecting society from the dangerous mental patient *and* protecting the patient from the dangers of his own mental illness. The professional, legal, and social legitimation of this double agency validates the mental health profession's core claim, that—regardless of whether the client is a voluntary or involuntary subject—the therapist is the patient's agent: "The physician seeks to liberate the patient from the chains of illness," explains Thomas G. Gutheil, professor of psychiatry at Harvard.[44] The claim that "commitment can be justified on the grounds of enhancing the individual's future freedom," is now psychiatric mantra.[45]

Psychiatric "Neutrality" and the "Funnel of Betrayal"

"As the prepatient may see it," wrote Erving Goffman in 1961, "the circuit of significant figures can function as a kind of betrayal funnel."[46] Today, the family's betrayal of the person they denominate as mentally ill is perceived as a self-sacrificial act, performed solely for the purpose of providing needed treatment for a "loved one."

For the supporters of psychiatric slavery, the proposition that oppressing the mental patient is a medical method for liberating him from his illness means that deceiving the patient is a higher form of morality. Indeed, psychiatrists sometimes acknowledge, with a kind of shame-faced pride, that they perjure themselves when they testify in court about a patient's dangerousness. Robert Miller, professor of psychiatry at the University of Wisconsin, states: "Thus it is easy to understand...why many psychiatrists reject the concept of a right to refuse treatment... Clinicians who wish to secure hospitalization for patients who are perceived to need it clinically, but who decline to accept it voluntarily, *must make allegations of future dangerousness in order to obtain authority to provide the needed treatment*...predictions of dangerousness are rarely challenged in commitment hearings."[47]

Thanks largely to the efforts of the National Alliance for the Mentally Ill (NAMI)—"a mental health advocacy organization that represents more than 200,000 families, consumers and providers across the country"—the funnel of betrayal has become a sophisticated technique of psychiatric slave-catching. NAMI, as will be evident, represents the interests of mental patients the same way the Ku Klux Klan represents the interests of black Americans. NAMI's website offers this recommendation for how to incriminate a "loved one" as "dangerous," in order to provide him with the "treatment" he "needs":

> Sometime, during the course of your loved one's illness, you may need the police... It is often difficult to get 911 to respond to your calls if you need someone to come & take your MI [mentally ill] relation to a hospital emergency room (ER)... When calling 911, the best way to get quick action is to say, "Violent EDP," or "Suicidal EDP." EDP stands for Emotionally Disturbed Person. This shows the operator that you know what you're talking about. Describe the danger very specifically. "He's a danger to himself "is not as good as "This morning my son said he was going to jump off the roof..." Also, give past history of violence. *This is especially important if the person is not acting up...* Realize that you & the cops are at cross purposes. You want them to take someone to the hospital. They don't want to do it... Say, "Officer, I understand your reluctance. Let me spell out for you the problems & the danger..." *While AMI/FAMI is not suggesting you do this, the fact is that some families have learned to "turn over the furniture" before calling the police...* If the police see furniture disturbed they will usually conclude that the person is imminently dangerous...[48]

Criminal law, based on a recognition of the intrinsically adversarial nature of the relationship between accused and accuser, separates the roles of prosecuting attorney and defense attorney. In contrast, mental health law, based on a denial of the intrinsically adversarial nature of the relationship between the person accused of mental illness and his accuser, combines and confuses the roles of prosecuting psychiatrist and defense psychiatrist: even when the psychiatrist imposes his intervention on a person against his will, mental health law defines the psychiatrist's role as serving the best interests of the patient.[49] No psychiatrist ever admits that he stands in an adversarial relationship to the person he calls a "patient." Instead, he claims that he is helping the patient or, in the court room, that he is an impartial expert testifying about matters of fact. "'Dream work' is working as a court-appointed expert," declares Gutheil. Seemingly unaware of the brutal narcissism that oozes from his remarks, he explains that such work is a dream "because usually the judge has some interest in your getting paid and wants to use you again. Also, being the center expert rather than partisan is for many people a very enjoyable experience."[50] Gutheil's profession of impartiality in the face of conflict places him squarely in the camp of the sinners Dante calls "opportunists" (in John Ciardi's classic translation).[51]

In the *Inferno*, Canto III, Dante (1265-1321) introduces the reader to "The Vestibule of Hell," the place where the souls of "the Opportunists" reside, and writes: "I, holding my head in horror, cried: 'Sweet Spirit, what souls are these who run through this black haze?' And he [Virgil] to me: 'These are the nearly soulless whose lives concluded neither blame nor praise. They are mixed here with that despicable corps of angels who were neither for God nor Satan, but only for themselves. The High Creator who scourged them from Heaven and Hell will not receive them since the wicked might feel glory over them... Mercy and Justice deny them even a name.'"[52]

Dante scholar John D. Sinclair calls these sinners "neutrals" instead of "opportunists," and considers them guilty of the vice of cowardice. He writes: "They have no need to die, for they 'never were alive.' They follow still, as they have always done, a meaningless shifting banner that never stands for anything because it never stands at all, a cause which is no cause but the changing magnet of the day."[53]

Mental health professionals deal with conflicts—between individuals, between individuals and institutions, and between the warring interests and impulses within individuals. By choosing to become mental health professionals—rather than, say, mathematicians or veterinarians—they *choose* to be parties to conflicts and must honestly acknowledge where they stand. If they do not, they deserve the fate that Dante believed awaits those who, faced with a conflict between Good and Evil, choose to remain neutral.

We do not accept the clergyman as an impartial expert in religious disputes. Yet, because we stubbornly *misdefine interpersonal and moral problems as medical problems,* we accept—indeed, embrace—the psychiatrist as an impartial expert in such disputes. The psychiatrist *chooses* to be involved in human conflicts and hence cannot avoid *choosing* sides. If he claims to be neutral—serving Health, Medicine, or Science—he perjures himself. And if we believe the perjurer, we deceive ourselves.

Conclusions

It is instructive to dwell for a moment on how diametrically our attitudes differ toward the needs of individuals for "clerical-religious help" (pastoral service), and their needs or alleged needs for "clinical-secular" help (mental health service). The American government provides no religious services for its civilian citizens (Congress excepted). Clergymen provide no involuntary religious services for atheists or others who do not voluntarily seek their ministrations.

They have no power to detain and imprison persons because they may be dangerous to themselves or others. Were a person to interpret such limitations on the powers of priests as "withholding religious services" from people who need them, he would be either dismissed as an ignoramus or disdained as an advocate of theocracy.

- American custom and law explicitly deprive the priest of legal authority to coerce people in the name of God.

- American custom and law explicitly authorize the psychiatrist to coerce people in the name of Mental Health.

Mental health professionals recoil from limiting their power to intefere "therapeutically" in the life of the patient, especially with respect to so-called suicide prevention.[54] This rejection of any *contractual limitation* on his actions vitiates what I regard as a precondition for maintaining the integrity of the therapist's role as agent of the patient. The therapist who professes to be the patient's agent cannot forcibly interfere in the patient's life. This kind of therapeutic self-restraint is now professionally censured as "withholding essential treatment" from the patient, and is rendered *de facto* illegal by tort law and, potentially, by criminal law as well.

In a free society, an adult can be coerced only for the benefit of society—by the police, if he is suspected of a crime, and by judge and jailer, if he is convicted of one. In such a society, an adult cannot be coerced for his own benefit—by educational authorities, to learn; by religious authorities, to be pious; or by medical authorities, to be treated. Yet, he can be coerced by psychiatric authorities, to be treated for mental illness.

To achieve a relationship between therapists and patients based on competence and trust—not credentials and power—the therapist-masters would have to relinquish their tools of legalized control and coercion. One of the most important of these tools is the pretense of possessing scientific "techniques" and "tests" that enable them to know the "best interests" of patients. This is a pretense to justify power over patients. Only after such and similar methods for maintaining the psychiatrist's dominance over patients are abolished can we begin to construct a framework of secular helpfulness respectful of personal dignity, liberty, and responsibility.

4

Justifying Psychiatric Slavery: "Dangerousness" as Disease

It is evident how much men love to deceive, and be deceived... And it is in vain to find fault with those arts of deceiving, wherein men find pleasure to be deceived.

—*John Locke (1690)*[1]

The welfare of the people in particular has always been the alibi of tyrants, and it provides the further advantage of giving the servants of tyranny a good conscience.

—*Albert Camus (1913-1960)*[2]

Before the Reformation and the Enlightenment, rulers enjoyed unlimited power over their subjects. But first in England, then in Switzerland and the United States, absolutist governments were replaced by limited governments. In England, Parliament limited the powers of the sovereign. In the United States, Congress limited the powers of the president. The result was the modern, Anglo-American concept of freedom: the individual has a right to life, liberty, and property, is presumed innocent of crime, and is subject to punishment for crimes, in conformity with due process.

The free society, as this idea is understood among political philosophers, rests on the principle that the citizen is a responsible adult possessing individual rights and owing duties to the community. In contrast, psychiatry, as a system of social practices, rests on the principle that the citizen is a potential mental patient who is, or might at any moment be, like an infant, requiring care and control. *Thus, the rule of law and the rule of psychiatric care are mutually incompatible.* The more we have of the one, the less we can have of the other.

Before the practice of mad-doctoring could become a recognized medical activity, it was necessary to rationalize depriving innocent

75

persons of property and liberty *outside the rules of the criminal justice system.* The new "science" of mad-doctoring fulfilled that role: it offered the idea of insanity as an illness that deprives the subject of reason, makes him child-like, renders him dangerous to himself and others, excuses him from punishment for his misbehavior, and renders him subject to control masquerading as care. This view of the madman and the methods for controlling him resonated with the classic legal principle of *parens patriae*: the insane person is like the infant and it is the duty of the state to care for him, for his own benefit as well as in the interest of the community.[3] The desired conclusion followed: as the person found guilty of a crime deserves to be punished (typically by confinement in prison), so the person diagnosed as mad needs to be treated (typically by confinement in an insane asylum).

Institutionalization and Deinstitutionalization

From 1800 to the 1950s, it was scientific dogma and conventional wisdom that madness is a medical malady and that mad persons must be forcibly detained and treated by medical specialists. In the late 1950s, the practice euphemistically called "mental hospitalization" was supplemented by the practice euphemistically called "deinstitutionalization." Forcible incarceration of the mental patient was replaced by mandatory eviction. Like institutionalization, deinstitutionalization required the use of state-sanctioned coercion. Why? Because, unlike the typical patient in a medical hospital who usually was a patient for a brief period and had a home and/or family to return to, the typical patient in a state mental hospital had no home of his own, his family did not want him, and, after years in the hospital, the institution became his home. In addition, far-reaching changes in the political-economic aspects of health care led to huge increases in the cost of maintaining patients in mental hospitals, providing a powerful economic incentive for closing those institutions.

As the policy of forcibly institutionalizing mental patients required justification, so did the policy of forcibly deinstitutionalizing them. This was accomplished by the claim that psychotropic drugs are effective treatments for mental illnesses and that the patient's best interests require that he be discharged from the hospital "to the least restrictive setting in the community." Again, the patients' preferences were ignored. Instead, decisions profoundly affecting their lives were imposed on them by force and declared to be in their own best interests: constraining mental patients by the *physically and socially most restrictive means possible* (long-term or life-long hospitalization) was replaced with constraining them by the *chemically and cognitively most restrictive means possible* (long-term or life-long drugging). Neither long-term mental hospitalization nor deinstitutionalization has anything to do with illness, treatment, or medicine. Both are legal and socio-economic policies for the psychiatric regulation of the lives of millions of Americans.[4]

Prior to deinstitutionalization, psychiatrists claimed that the best treatment for seriously ill mental patients was long-term hospitalization, combined with insulin shock or electric shock. Since deinstitutionalization, they claim that the best treatment for them is short-term hospitalization, combined with antipsychotic medication and community placement. Both claims are pseudoscientific fables, concealing heartless bureaucratic-psychiatric policies of stigmatizing, disabling, segregating, and storing unwanted persons.[5]

In 1955, Daniel Blain, the medical director of the American Psychiatric Association, declared: "The 750,000 patients now in this country's mental hospitals would soon be returned to the community, *cured*."[6] The reality was rather different: "In New York State," wrote a British reporter, "a large number of psychiatric patients were recently thrown out of large institutions, almost literally overnight, and left to wander the city streets... Yet when winter comes, those very people are rounded up and herded into huge warehouses, not much different from the workhouses of old, where they are 'kept' for the winter."[7]

Actually, after treatment with neuroleptic drugs and deinstitutionalization, most mental patients are worse off than they were before: the problems in living that led to their categorization as mentally ill are not remedied; in many cases their troubles are compounded by tardive dyskinesia, a disfiguring neurological disease caused by neuroleptic drugs; and most patients continue to depend on family or society for food and shelter.

Confronting Preventive Psychiatric Detention

Our love of freedom requires that laws protect the citizen accused of lawbreaking, otherwise we run the risk of the government overpowering the citizen. Our need for safety requires that laws protect the community, otherwise we run the risk of individuals harming each other and destroying society. This is a dilemma every modern society must face.[8]

Regardless of what it is called, depriving innocent persons of liberty with the sanction of the law (justified as the prevention of harm to self or others) is *preventive detention.* It is impossible to understand our love-hate relationship with this social sanction unless we appreciate that modern states are therapeutic states, that is, societies in which medicine and the state are united in much the same way as church and state had been united (and still are in some parts of the world).[9] This is why we *reject preventive detention of the innocent as violation of due process, but embrace preventive detention of the insane as medical treatment and/or public health measure.* The result is psychiatry, ostensibly a medical specialty, *committed to the principle of preventively imprisoning innocent persons called "patients"*—to protect them and society from the dangers of "mental illness." Americans are unwilling to confront the following facts:

- No one can prevent a person who truly wants to kill himself from doing so.

- No one can prevent a person from assaulting or killing others if he is prepared to sacrifice his life to achieve his goal, as the example of suicide-bombers tragically demonstrates.

- There is no evidence that suicide prevention programs are effective.

- "It is the official policy of the American Psychiatric Association that psychiatrists are incapable of predicting dangerousness."[10]

None of this deters psychiatrists from engaging in the lucrative business of trying to prevent dangerousness, or dissuades law enforcement authorities, the media, and the public from embracing and promoting this counterproductive, immoral practice. Routinely, the mere suspicion of mental illness as a cause of suicide justifies outrageous police behavior, such as the following: "A Virginia court has issued a blistering rebuke of the Fairfax County police department's tactical unit, saying its black-clad officers illegally burst into homes—in one instance repeatedly shooting a man they were trying to take in for mental treatment."[11]

The fact that we accept suicide prevention as a justification for civil commitment is *prima facie* evidence that *the most important function of involuntary mental hospitalization is preventive detention.* The true motive for the use of psychiatric force is not protection from dangerousness, but the desire to get rid of unwanted persons, especially family members. In the United States, the die was

cast a hundred and fifty years ago. Ever since then, American custom and law have endorsed the practice of locking up people in
mental hospitals, even if no one really believes they are mentally ill
or dangerous:

- In 1851, the State of Illinois enacted a statute specifying that "married
  women...may be received and detained at the hospital on the request
  of the husband of the woman...without the evidence of insanity or
  distraction required in other cases."[12]

- In 1997, in *Kansas v. Leroy Hendricks,* the U. S. Supreme Court declared: "States have a right to use psychiatric hospitals to confine
  certain sex offenders once they have completed their prison terms,
  even if those offenders do not meet mental illness commitment criteria."[13]

- In February 2000, Wisconsin's oldest prison inmate, a ninety-five-
  year-old man, was "resentenced" as a sexual predator. A psychologist
  "testified for the state and said psychological tests performed on
  Ellefson indicated if he was given a chance, he would commit a [sex]
  crime... After only minutes of deliberation, the jury found that Ellef J.
  Ellefson should be committed for mental treatment under the sexual
  predator law."[14]

The Pretense that Coercion is Care

Although some commentators on mental health law acknowledge
that defining involuntary mental hospitalization as treatment is a fraud,
they accept the reality of mental illness and the legitimacy of psychiatric coercions and excuses.

- Alan A. Stone, professor of law and psychiatry at Harvard University
  and a former president of the APA: "Psychiatry, by calling custodial
  confinement 'treatment,' gave legitimacy to the practice of locking
  people up for the rest of their lives whether they were dangerous or
  not."[15]

- John Q. La Fond and Mary L. Durham, a law professor and social
  scientist in Washington: "Momentum for expanding control over the
  mentally ill is growing at a rapid rate. Increasingly, psychiatrists and
  other mental health professionals...serve as agents of social control,
  whether or not they are comfortable with that assignment."[16]

- John J. Sandford, a British forensic psychiatrist: "The preventive detention of those with untreatable mental disorders is already widely
  practiced in England. Under the Mental Health Act (1983) people...[are]
  detained indefinitely in hospital regardless of response to treatment

and on grounds of risk to self as well as others. Secure and open psychiatric hospitals are full of such patients."[17]

- An editorial in the *British Medical Journal*: "The growing pressures on them [psychiatrists] to deliver public protection was perhaps inevitable, given the rise of biopsychomedical paradigms as explanations for the vicissitudes of life in modern Western society. Psychiatrists have played their part by assuming the authority to explain, categorize, manage, and prognose in situations where well defined disease (arguably their only clearcut remit) was not present."[18]

Dissatisfied with current mental health laws in the United Kingdom, Szmukler and Holloway, two British psychiatrists, suggest repealing the U.K. Mental Health Act of 1983 and replacing it with "some kind of dangerousness legislation... If the person is mentally ill and treatment will eliminate or reduce the risk, a psychiatric disposal may be appropriate... Psychiatrists [would] be required only to treat people detained by a court."[19] Disingenuously, they then ask: "Why should different rules govern society's response to dangerous mentally disordered persons compared to dangerous non-mentally disordered persons?"[20] The answer is obvious. Because psychiatrists have taught the public to view the "mentally disordered person" as less than a full-fledged person, a being unable to control his own behavior. Hence, we regard it as our (common sense) duty to protect the "patient" from harming himself or others; and call depriving him of liberty "treatment." In contrast, we view the "non-mentally disordered person" as a full-fledged person, responsible for his behavior. Hence, we do not regard it as our (common sense) duty to protect him from harming himself or others; and call depriving him of liberty "punishment."

It is a basic tenet of English and American law that it is morally wicked to deprive an innocent person of liberty, even in the service of a "good cause." It is better, we say, to let a hundred guilty men go free than to imprison a single innocent person. The opposite rule governs "psychiatric ethics": "[I] would rather detain nine people unnecessarily than discharge one who went on to harm a member of the public," proclaimed a psychiatrist on prime time British TV.[21] The contrast between the presumption of innocence in the criminal justice system and the presumption of mental illness in the mental health system epitomizes the incompatibility between psychiatric preventive detention and the rule of law. The diaphanous veil of due process, laid over the imposition of psychiatric diagnoses and the enforcement of psychiatric sanctions, masks the utter lawlessness of these methods of social control.

If the centuries-old debate about psychiatric coercion teaches us anything, it is that we deceive ourselves if we pay attention to what lawyers and psychiatrists say instead of what they do. Regardless of what it is called, civil commitment is preventive detention masquerading as a medical procedure: it is the psychiatric removal and segregation of society's unwanted.

Reconsidering the Dangerousness of Mental Illness

In the ancient world, the idea of madness was associated with divine inspiration and wisdom, not dangerousness and dementia. The bracketing of madness with dangerousness is a modern invention, roughly contemporaneous with the birth of mad-doctoring as preventive detention and the concept of insanity as illness. The nature and magnitude of the danger allegedly intrinsic to mental illness and the best methods for coping with it form a large part of the history of psychiatry. However, since "mental illness" is not contagious, "it" cannot pose a danger as a disease.[22] The association between mental illness and dangerousness is a consequence of managing lawlessness as if it were a contagious disease, and partly a matter of semantics, that is, calling criminals "sick."

Mad dogs are nasty animals that are perhaps infected with the contagious illness called "rabies." Mad cows are sick animals that suffer from the infectious illness called "bovine spongiform encephalitis." Prior to World War II, many people called "mad" suffered from the consequence of the contagious illness syphilis, called neurosyphilis.

Calling a person "mad" implies both that he is angry and that he suffers from a disease. Persons who rave and rant as well as persons who commit violent crimes are often said to be mad or insane or mentally ill. There is a kind of tautological truth in this bracketing, inasmuch as individuals who engage in violent and lawless acts are often diagnosed as mentally ill and treated as mental patients. No medical disease has the kind of linguistic and legal linkage with aggression and lawlessness associated with mental illness. When epilepsy was considered a mental illness, it was believed to be a cause of crime, especially assault and murder; when it became a brain disease, its association with dangerousness disappeared.[23]

The Ethics of Psychiatric Slavery: Protection from Dangerousness

The twin ideas that crime is disease and that punishment is treatment are psychiatry's old hat. Classic psychiatric practice is synonymous with incarceration regardless of guilt or innocence. Classic psychiatric theory is synonymous with abolishing the distinction between crime and disease.

In 1907, the French psychiatrist Joseph Grasset declared: "The obligation of *medical surveillance and treatment after the expiration of the punishment should be incorporated in the law*... the accused at the expiration of his punishment is looked upon as a sick person... Yes, we really have a patient on our hands, but a patient who has been and who still can be harmful to society. *It is therefore necessary to nurse him by force.*"[24]

In 1968, famed American psychiatrist Karl Menninger (1893-1990) opined: "When the community begins to look upon the expression of aggression as the symptom of an illness or as indicative of illness, it will be because it believes doctors can do something to correct such a condition... Do I believe there is effective treatment for offenders? Most certainly and definitely I do."[25]

The psychiatrization of crime and punishment has recently been re-embraced, in both the United Kingdom and the United States, as if it represented enlightened social policy, based on fresh scientific insights into the workings of the mind-brain. In 1999, United Kingdom Home Secretary Jack Straw announced "the immediate introduction of measures to keep track of people who are still judged to be a risk to society when they are released from prison or a mental-health institution."[26] By May 2000, Parliament was considering "Proposals to lock up mentally ill people perceived as a danger to society, even if they have not committed a crime... The MPs...called for a broader medical definition to include the 'management' of potentially dangerous patients."[27] In July, 2001, *The Sunday Times* (London) reported: "An elite team of detectives and psychiatrists is being set up by police to target would-be killers and stop them before they commit murder... Information [will be obtained] from mental health agencies and social security and hospital records... After compiling a list of possible killers, psychologists will draw up a profile to establish whether their pattern of behavior makes them a 'real danger.'"[28]

Straw was hoisting psychiatrists by their own petard. Answering questions in Parliament, he insisted "that the care of *untreatable de-*

tainees would indeed fall within the health, and not the judicial, service: 'The medical profession and mental health tribunals already have substantial experience of depriving people of their liberty where individuals with severe personality disorders are classified as treatable... If it is right to detain people who have treatable severe personality disorders, why on earth is it wrong to detain people who are regarded as untreatable but who continue to pose exactly the same or worse risk to the public?'"[29] Straw might have added that viewing insanity as incurable never stopped psychiatrists from incarcerating the insane.

A senior member of the Royal College of Psychiatrists protested that the incarceration of individuals with personality disorders "must be done openly as *preventive detention for the protection of the public, and not dressed up as 'these poor people are sick.'*"[30] It is too late for that. The entire psychiatric slave system rests squarely on the tradition-sanctioned deception that imprisonment is treatment. Under British law, innocent individuals can be imprisoned *only* under the guise of needing psychiatric treatment for their illness.

Some psychiatrists recognize that the government is using them immorally, turning them into agents of social control, pure and simple. Nigel Eastman, senior lecturer in forensic psychiatry at St. George's Hospital Medical School in London, writes:

> The core public policy objective is clearly public protection... There will be an indeterminate but reviewable order imposed by a court on evidence from psychiatrists (and perhaps psychologists) which will remain in place so long as the person is deemed, again on expert evidence, sufficiently dangerous to warrant it... The order will also apply to the untreatable... Why make the new order a health order at all? ...[Because] a "health order" is the only route available to the government to secure its goal. As a result, doctors (and perhaps psychologists) will be required to "diagnose" the new legal concept of severe personality disorder... the effect of such recommendations will often not be treatment but punishment, or preventive detention... *Under the new order, both the convicted and the unconvicted, will be detained in a specialist secure service which must necessarily be legally a "hospital," since unconvicted people cannot be imprisoned...* The fragility of the distinction between public health psychiatry and crime prevention has never before been so starkly represented.[31]

Perhaps without intending to, Eastman succeeds in exposing the therapeutic state and the pharmacratic regulations on which it depends in all their naked goriness. Clearly, we are heading toward the complete disappearance of free psychiatry, that is, a psychiatry serving the patient and only the patient.

Dangerousness Is Not A Disease

The idea of dangerousness as a treatable illness is the keystone of the psychiatric slave system, much as *the idea of insanity as an illness* is the keystone of psychiatry as a medical specialty.[32] Associating dangerousness with mental illness is necessary for the maintenance of psychiatric slavery, just as associating racial inferiority with the Negro race was necessary for the maintenance of chattel slavery. Moreover, nothing is easier than to conduct a so-called psychiatric study and show that there is a positive correlation between one or another undesirable behavior and mental illness. Homelessness, drunkenness, drug abuse, poverty, divorce, suicide, murder, street crime, have all been shown to be "associated with" or "caused by" mental illness. What do such studies show? Whatever the "researcher" wants to prove.

From a scientific point of view, every study investigating the association between mental illness and dangerousness is a hoax. In the first place, there is no objective method for identifying whether or not a person is mentally ill; secondly, psychiatric researchers are not interested in "finding things out,"[33] they are interested in setting and justifying policies.[34] It is not surprising, therefore, that some studies show that mental patients are more dangerous than are normal persons, and other studies show they are not; some studies show that psychiatrists can predict patient dangerousness, others that they cannot do so.

Robert I. Simon, professor of psychiatry at Georgetown University School of Medicine, asserts: "Studies show that...predicting violence for an individual cannot be done accurately."[35] A Swedish psychiatrist reports that "at most, 100 serious assaults a year in Sweden were committed by patients who had been discharged during the previous year from involuntary psychiatric treatment—that is, less than 1% of all patients discharged"; and concludes that "the ratio of correct to false positive predictions of assault would be about 1 in 30. ...predictions of violence and restraining psychiatric patients into more custodial care is not only useless for society but bears extremely high cost for those many patients falsely predicted to become violent."[36] In contrast, a British psychiatrist claims that the profession of psychiatry "was slow to recognize the statistical association between schizophrenia and violence."[37] As we have seen, this is not true: mental illness has always been associated with dangerousness.

Today, it is conventional wisdom to believe that persons who deliberately injure or kill themselves or others are mentally ill. *Ergo,* mentally ill persons are more likely to injure or kill themselves or others than are normal persons. True, persons incarcerated in mental hospitals or discharged from them often attack others, especially persons whom they hold responsible for depriving them of liberty. Psychiatrists interpret the attackers' behavior as further evidence that they are mentally ill. I interpret it as a form of revenge or slave revolt. Attacks on mental health personnel by mental patients is strong evidence that mental health professionals cannot predict patient dangerousness.

Conclusions

Psychiatric coercion is both the solution for, and a cause of, the problem of the dangerousness of the mental patient. The threat of psychiatric coercion is often the precipitating cause of assault, murder, and suicide.

It is intrinsic to the nature of the master-slave relationship that the slave poses a permanent threat to his oppressor. In the antebellum South, it was received wisdom that "The negro, as a general rule, is mendacious."[38] In the United States today, it is received wisdom that the mental patient is dangerous.

The person who threatens to harm or kill someone (other than himself) violates criminal law and his behavior could be controlled by penal sanctions, without recourse to preventive psychiatric detention.

Psychiatrists regularly make contradictory claims about their ability to predict patient dangerousness, according to their particular needs. If psychiatrists could predict such behavior, they would not so frequently be the victims of assaults by their own patients.[39]

None of the ideas and observations discussed in this chapter are new. In 1898, an editorial in the *Journal of Mental Science* declared: "The public should be instructed that the annually recurring and possibly increasing horrors from the crimes of 'lunatics at large' are the price it pays, under the existing lunacy law, *for protection from an illusory danger to the 'liberty of the subject.'"[40]

If the subject is a slave or incarcerated mental patient, liberty is the most important thing in his life.

5

Jim Crow Psychiatry I:
The Psychiatric Will and Its Enemies

The movement of the progressive societies has hitherto been a movement *from Status to Contract.*

—*Henry Sumner Maine (1822-1888)[1]*

Morality consists in the recognition of individual personality wherever it appears. Moreover, personality is so far sacrosanct that no man has either a right or a duty to promote the moral perfection of another: we may promote the "happiness" of others, but we cannot promote their "good" without destroying their "freedom," which is the condition of moral goodness.

—*Michael Oakeshott (1901-1992)[2]*

Jim Crow laws, named after an antebellum minstrel show character, were post-Civil War statutes passed by the legislatures of the Southern states to create a racial caste system. The war and its aftermath intensified, rather than diminished, white supremacist views. As a result, laws were enacted that legitimized discriminatory social practices aimed at excluding blacks from educational and employment opportunities and deprived them of many rights outwardly granted them by emancipation. In 1896, in its infamous ruling in *Plessy v. Ferguson*, the Supreme Court sanctified the ideology of Jim Crow by constitutionalizing the principle of "separate but equal." The legal structure of segregation was not dismantled until the enactment of civil rights legislation sixty years later.[3] And even that was not the end of the matter. "The voting rights act of 1965 and desegregation did not erase racism and did not even remove much de facto segregation."[4] Law or no law, people avoid others whom they fear or dislike.

Psychiatrists have always maintained that involuntary mental patients are ill and hospitalized exactly as the physician's voluntary medical patients are ill and hospitalized. This is a brazen falsehood which, since the advent of psychotropic drugs in the late 1950s, psychiatrists have tried, with considerable success, to transform into politically correct "truth." Politicians and medical professionals, jurists and journalists, lawyers and the public believe, or pretend to believe, that "mental illness is like any other illness." The result is a plethora of special mental health laws legitimating the twin principles of Jim Crow psychiatry: for mental illness, "identical-but-different"; for the mentally ill person, "unequal and separate."

Ostensibly liberated by the Thirteenth Amendment, blacks were declared to be the equals of whites, but were separated from them socially and were treated differently by the legal system. Psychiatric patients are declared the equals of medical patients, but are separated from them socially and are treated differently by the legal system. For example, medical patients are presumed to be competent: they can execute medical advance directives and reject medical treatment. Psychiatric patients are presumed to be incompetent: they cannot execute a true psychiatric advance directive (PAD) and reject psychiatric treatment. "Mental illness," explains Paul S. Appelbaum, "by definition calls the soundness of the mind—and therefore the legal competence—of the actor into question. This perspective ...accounts (in part) for the traditional assumption that *consent for treatment need not be obtained from the mentally ill*."[5]

Threats to the legitimacy of the psychiatric principle of "identical-but-different" provoke howls of indignation from psychiatric supremacists. Responding to a ruling by a Massachusetts court limiting the psychiatrist's discretion to forcibly drug mental hospital patients, Thomas G. Gutheil declared: "[This ruling] clearly illustrates the failure of the legal mind to grasp clinical realities... *The physician seeks to liberate the patient from the chains of illness; the judge, from the chains of treatment*."[6] After more than two hundred years of psychiatric "reforms," it ought to be obvious that as long as the basic premises of psychiatry enjoy legitimacy, persons called "mental patients" will remain disfranchised, if not in one way, then in another.

Many blacks were worse off under Jim Crow laws than they had been under slavery. Now many mental patients are worse off than they had been before they "enjoyed" the "benefits" of the new rights granted them. The more scrupulously the mental patient's status is regulated by law, the more he loses the protection of the legal system, and the more that system is used as an instrument for his destruction in the name of "therapy." At the 1980 annual meeting of the American Academy of Psychiatry and Law, two psychiatrists from Washington, D.C.'s Saint Elizabeths Hospital declared their "commitment to freedom": "Is a stuporous catatonic freer successfully refusing fluphenazine, or is his life freer if given the fluphenazine involuntarily? ...We would submit that commitment can be justified on the grounds of *enhancing the individual's future freedom.*"[7] These psychiatrists are untroubled about attributing the capacity to "successfully refuse" psychiatric medication to a person they characterize as "a stuporous catatonic"; also, they are unconcerned about the contradiction inherent in depriving a person of liberty in order to liberate him.

Psychiatric News, the APA's bimonthly newspaper, uses the language of liberty to defend psychiatric despotism: "Psychiatry [stands] fully behind the principle *that psychiatric institutions be utilized for increasing the freedom of the mentally ill.*"[8]

The crime committed against the liberty of the psychiatric patient is further illustrated by the following: A medical patient has the legal right to refuse surgical or pharmacological therapy even when such treatment is unequivocally beneficial, curative, or even life-saving; yet, a psychiatric patient cannot refuse treatment, even when there is no evidence that it will improve, let alone cure, his condition. In effect, the state recognizes the medical patient's right to *certain* death (by refusing effective treatment for a fatal disease), but denies the mental patient's right to *potential* death (by committing suicide).

For the slave owner, the idea of the black slave's (or colonized person's) self-determination was anathema—an insult to his obligation as a white man ("the white man's burden"). For the psychiatrist, the idea of the mental patient's self-determination is anathema—an insult to his obligation as a healer ("the psychiatrist's burden"). That is why psychiatric advance directives force mental patients to sit at the back of the bus driven by medical ethicists enlightened by the new psychiatry.

The Psychiatric Will (PW)

Unlike the medical or surgical physician, the psychiatric physician has many patients who do not want to be patients at all. They want to be left alone, unmolested by the attentions "their" doctors foist on them against their bitterest protests. It is important to keep in mind that, for centuries, the only kinds of patients that mad-doctors, alienists, and psychiatrists had were persons who did not want to be patients.

Although the clientele of the typical contemporary psychiatrist includes voluntary patients, he also has involuntary patients; moreover, he continues to have the right and the duty to diagnose, detain, and treat people against their will, *including individuals who seek his services voluntarily*. In short, mental illnesses differ from bodily illnesses, mental patients differ from medical patients, and psychiatric physicians differ from other physicians. Almost a hundred years ago, Karl Jaspers—famed psychiatrist-turned-philosopher—noted that this elementary fact sets psychiatry apart from medicine and renders the "rational treatment" of mental patients moot. "Admission to hospital," he wrote, "often takes place against the will of the patient and therefore the psychiatrist finds himself in a different relation to his patient than other doctors... Rational treatment is not really an attainable goal as regards the large majority of mental patients in the strict sense."[9] Jurists and psychiatrists refuse to acknowledge this embarrassing fact and its far-reaching implications.

The basic virtue or wickedness of slavery—depending on one's point of view—was *altruistic coercive paternalism*. The same is true for psychiatry. Like the slave owner, the psychiatrist denies that conflict between him and his involuntary patient is intrinsic to their relationship; he insists that if the patient were rational, he would agree that he is mentally ill and needs precisely the treatment that the psychiatrist is imposing on him.

The psychiatrist maintains that he is the involuntary mental patient's agent, representing the patient's own best interests. I maintain that, by definition, the interests of the coercive psychiatrist and of the involuntary mental patient conflict. The coercive psychiatrist is the involuntary patient's adversary, not his ally.

The altruistic-paternalistic premise infects all mental health laws, which differ from other laws. One of the principal differences between civil and criminal laws is that violations of the former are typically punished by deprivation of property (fine), whereas violations of the latter (unless minor) are typically punished by deprivation of liberty (imprisonment). *De jure*, mental health laws are civil laws. *De facto*, they are criminal laws: their violation results in deprivation of liberty, called "hospitalization." This ruse makes the mental patient utterly defenseless against his adversaries, officially defined and recognized as his allies. Unlike all other deprivations of liberty, deprivation of liberty under psychiatric auspices is considered "treatment."

For centuries, the law treated all persons deemed "certifiable" as, *ipso facto*, mentally incompetent: the subject was placed in the status of a child—dependent on a parent or parent surrogate—and the psychiatrist, as agent of the state, was placed in the role of his parent, with a duty to care for him *(parens patriae)*. This psychiatric style remained essentially unchanged until the 1960s, when, under the influence of the civil rights movement, psychiatrists and some former mental patients began to demand rights for mental patients, *qua mental patients*. This misguided strategy quickly led to the legal and psychiatric acknowledgment of what had always been obvious, namely, that most mental patients are not, and have never been, mentally or legally incompetent. At the same time, the strategy represented another fatally flawed attempt at so-called mental health law reform: the "reform" rested on the fundamentally deceptive and false claim that mental illness is the name of a class of objectively identifiable, legitimate diseases. However, since it is the state that deprives individuals of their liberty, in their own best interest as mental patients, the state cannot also protect them from the loss of their rights which the state approves as an indispensable element of their medical treatment.

Modern psychiatric opinion holds that "even being under a commitment does not in and of itself make a person incompetent."[10] The view that *some time during his life* the involuntarily hospitalized mental patient is a competent adult, able and entitled to make decisions for himself, framed the context in which, in 1982, I proposed a new legal-psychiatric instrument, the Psychiatric Will (PW).[11] Specifically, the instrument was intended, as the paper's subtitle indicated, to provide "a new mechanism for protecting persons against 'psychosis' and psychiatry." More broadly, its aim was to clarify, mediate, and eventually resolve the conflict between the coercive psychiatrist and the coerced patient and, generally, between persons who support coercions in the name of mental health as therapeutic ("psychiatric protectionists"), and those who oppose such practices and seek to place psychiatric relations on a contractual basis ("psychiatric voluntarists").

The Anatomy of the Psychiatric Will

The avowed desires of patients and doctors conflict far more often in psychiatry than in any other branch of medical practice. Unlike medical interventions, psychiatric interventions are routinely imposed on patients against their will. Hence, the person who voluntarily consults a psychiatrist runs the risk of becoming the subject of unwanted psychiatric interventions. Accordingly, advance directives are most important and most useful for potential psychiatric patients.

The contact between patient and doctor is dangerous for the psychiatrist as well. The psychiatrist who gives an appointment to a person-as-patient is at risk of becoming the defendant in a malpractice suit he cannot win. Thus, like the medical advance directive, which protects both patient and doctor, the psychiatric will, too, would protect both patient and doctor. Prospectively consenting to or refusing involuntary psychiatric interventions, the PW would constitute a legally binding agreement between the potential psychiatric patient and his potential psychiatrist: the contract would protect the patient from becoming the victim of unwanted psychiatric coercion, and the psychiatrist from becoming the victim of malpractice litigation as long as he obeys the terms of the contract.[12] While the protective function of the PW for the patient is obvious, its protective function for the psychiatrist may be less clear. I shall briefly discuss each.

As matters stand, the person with a psychiatric diagnosis deemed to have diminished decisional capacity is administered psychiatric treatment against his will. He has no right to reject such "treatment": the very act of rejecting psychiatric help is now interpreted as a symptom of mental illness, a manifestation of dangerousness to self or others, and a justification for involuntary treatment. In short, the PW offers individuals the option to prospectively choose to receive or reject involuntary psychiatric treatment. At the same time, it preserves the psychiatrists' ability to administer involuntary treatments, provided individuals request such interventions in their psychiatric wills.

The PW also protects the psychiatrist endangered by his so-called special relationship with the patient. Having to act as both physician and guardian, the psychiatrist may be held legally liable for the deleterious consequences of both coercing and not coercing the patient. The PW would protect him from both contingencies. The following hypothetical, but typical, scenario illustrates the psychiatrist's predicament.

> A middle-aged, married executive, with three children all under ten years of age, becomes disenchanted with his wife, falls in love with his young secretary, has an affair with her, and contemplates divorce. Overcome with conflict over the existential complexities in which he is enmeshed, he becomes depressed, confesses all to his wife, and hints that perhaps it would be best for everyone if he killed himself. She persuades him to see a psychiatrist. The psychiatrist diagnoses the husband as suffering from depression, prescribes antidepressant medication, and asks him to return a week later. Reluctantly, the patient returns. The psychiatrist concludes that the patient's depression has worsened, recommends immediate psychiatric hospitalization, and informs both the patient and his wife that the danger of suicide is the reason for this recommendation.

Scenario 1: The patient requests permission to go to his office to take care of some important business matters before checking into the hospital. He leaves, goes to his office, and shoots himself in the head. The wound is not fatal, but causes extensive brain damage that renders him a complete invalid. The patient's wife sues the psychiatrist, charging him with medical negligence for not admitting her husband directly to the hospital. She obtains a substantial settlement.

Scenario 2: The psychiatrist prevents the patient from leaving his office and commits him. The patient conducts himself well in the hospital and is quickly released. He then sues the psychiatrist for false imprisonment and damages to his business and reputation suffered as a result of the psychiatrist's action. He, too, obtains a substantial settlement.

The Psychiatric Will In Action

How would the PW actually work? Like the last will that becomes operative only after the testator is declared dead, the psychiatric will would become operative only after the subject is declared mentally ill and decisionally impaired or incapacitated.

Some persons fear the dangers of psychosis: they could use the PW to protect themselves from it, stipulating the kind of involuntary treatment they are willing to receive if they become mentally ill and lose their decisional capacity. Others fear the dangers of psychiatry: they could use the PW to protect themselves from it, stipulating their wish to reject psychiatric assistance and be held accountable for their behavior. The psychiatric will would thus protect the right of every adult—considered competent by mental health professionals at the time of executing the directive—to receive or reject future psychiatric services. The PW would be especially useful for persons who have undergone one or more episodes of involuntary psychiatric treatment. Having had first-hand experience with psychiatric interventions, they would be in a position to know what sorts of psychiatric assistance they may want to receive or reject in the future, should they be deemed to require psychiatric care.

To be valid, the psychiatric will, like the last will, would have to be executed by a person considered to be legally competent at the time of its execution. This criterion is met, *a priori*, by adults without a criminal record, living independently and not receiving psychiatric treatment; by adults receiving psychiatric treatment as outpatients; and by adults discharged from psychiatric hospitals and living on their own. Since such persons are considered capable of making contracts unrelated to psychiatric matters, and since courts grant even *"mentally ill people under guardianship"* the right to vote in state and federal elections, it is difficult to see on what grounds people could be denied the right to execute a valid psychiatric will.[13]

As a practical matter, there could be two different versions or implementations of the PW. In the weak version, the person would be subject to involuntary psychiatric interventions unless he affirmatively rejects them. In the strong version, the person would be spared involuntary psychiatric interventions unless he affirmatively requests them.

In principle, the strong version of the PW is more attractive. In practice, because of our long tradition of coercive psychiatric paternalism, the weak version may be more acceptable. In any case, no one executing a psychiatric will would have to receive or reject psychiatric interventions in their totality. Some persons might wish to permit coerced hospitalization, but prohibit treatment by drugs or electroshock. Others might wish to permit coerced drug therapy, but prohibit involuntary hospitalization. To be sure, the contemporary psychiatrist would reject a mental health policy that would allow a person to choose involuntary mental hospitalization but reject psychiatric treatment. The psychiatrists would feel, not without justification, that if a patient is permitted to stay in the hospital without treatment, the patient, not the doctor, uses the facility. Psychiatrists probably would look more favorably on the second option: authorizing involuntary drugging without hospitalization would not so radically threaten the psychiatrist's frail self-concept as a real doctor.

The options provided by the PW ought to satisfy the demands of both psychiatric protectionists and psychiatric voluntarists. Protectionists could not, in good faith, object to being frustrated in their therapeutic efforts by persons competent to make binding decisions about their future who choose to prohibit unauthorized psychiatric assistance. Similarly, voluntarists could not, in good faith, object to being frustrated in their libertarian efforts by persons competent to make binding decisions about their future who choose to authorize their own psychiatric tutelage. Adopting the PW—letting people choose to receive or reject psychiatric care, including coercive care, as they deem right—might put an end to the dispute about involuntary psychiatric interventions.

If a person believes that, if he were declared decisionally impaired and in need of psychiatric treatment, the psychiatrist's coercive intervention would serve his own best interests, then he has no particular need for a PW. However, if he believes that, in such a situation, the psychiatrist's coercive intervention would not serve his own best interests, then nothing short of repealing mental health laws could protect him from becoming the victim of psychiatric violence, justified as treatment for mental illness. *Mutatis mutandis*, nothing short of holding the person guilty of lawlessness, regardless of his having an alleged mental illness, could protect innocent people from becoming the victims of crimes by mental patients, for which the patients are not held accountable because their bad behaviors are attributed to mental illness.

In summary, the PW I proposed would: 1) preserve the ability of psychiatrists to administer, and of patients to receive, involuntary treatment, provided the patients request such treatment in their PWs; 2) compel lawyers and psychiatrists to confront and transcend the misleading conflation of mental illness with decisional impairment and legal incompetence; and 3) facilitate the gradual emancipation of the mental patient from psychiatric tutelage and the eventual abolition of psychiatric slavery. Patient and doctor together could use the PW to transform a potentially coercive relationship into a consensual one; or the patient could use it to avoid psychiatric coercions and assume full legal responsibility for the consequences of his behavior. Thus, there would be "parity" with respect to patients' rights to forego treatment: they would have the same rights to reject treatment for medical illness and mental illness.

Criticisms of the Psychiatric Will

The psychiatrist's *a priori* rejection of the person's right to self-determination explains why—despite, or rather because of, the obvious advantages of a genuine PW for both mental patient and psychiatrist—psychiatrists not only reject it but turn it into a fresh instrument of psychiatric domination. To the best of my knowledge, not a single American psychiatrist supports the PW, that is, a psychiatric advance directive similar to a medical advance directive. At the same time, many American psychiatrists (and lawyers as well) support a perverted form of the PW, that is, a legal instrument giving mental patients the fake choice to prospectively request psychiatric coercions, but denying them the real choice to prospectively reject such measures.[14]

Rejecting and Perverting the Psychiatric Will

How do psychiatrists rationalize their objections to the PW? Some oppose it on the ground that my "equation of illness with an organic base is stiflingly narrow."[15] However, the usefulness of the PW does not depend on the definition of illness. As the validity of the last will is independent of the nature or kind of property the testator wishes to bequeath, so the value of the PW is independent of the nature of "mental illness" or the effectiveness of any particular psychiatric intervention. Being the victim of religious persecution does not require that there be a God; similarly, being the victim of psychiatric oppression does not require that there be mental illness.

Other psychiatrists condemn the PW as an instrument for "turning back the clock" on the psychiatric profession's "commitment to freedom": "The average length of stay in state mental hospitals is less than one month. The average length of stay in prisons is measured in months and years... How does this promote liberty and freedom?"[16] Sometimes the opposite is the case. John W. Hinckley, Jr. has been "hospitalized" since 1981.[17] It is revealing of the psychiatric mindset that a psychiatrist casually compares the average length of stay of innocent persons in mental hospitals with the average length of stay of persons convicted of crimes in prisons, instead of with the average length of stay of physically ill patients in medical hospitals. By comparing confinement in a mental hospital with confinement in a prison, the writer conflates doctors and jailers, hospitals and prisons, innocent patients and guilty convicts, and tacitly admits that mental hospitalization is *de facto* imprisonment. Illness, *qua* illness, is never a justification for depriving the ill person of liberty. An institution the person cannot leave, legally or physically, should not be called a "hospital."

It is a truism that no social policy is free of costs, or "externalities," as economists call it. One of the externalities of the PW is that a person deemed committable by conventional criteria but left at liberty might harm others, imposing personal and financial costs on families, insurance companies, and the state. However, the present policy of involuntarily hospitalizing and/or treating countless dangerous as well as non-dangerous persons also entails great personal and financial cost to families, insurance companies, and the state. It is by no means obvious which is more costly—maintaining psychiatric slavery or abolishing it. In any case, in Anglo-American political philosophy, individual liberty is supposed to be priceless, dramatically reflected in the enormous cost born by the taxpayer for prosecuting each death penalty case.

A genuine psychiatric advance directive (PAD), like a medical advance directive, must cut both ways. If the PAD lets the subject request involuntary psychiatric intervention but doesn't let him reject such intervention, then it is not a real advance directive but a wicked trick.

As we have seen, it is precisely the choice to request *and* reject psychiatric interventions that psychiatrists are unwilling to offer *anyone*, let alone persons who have ever been diagnosed as mentally ill; and it is precisely because my version of the PW offers *everyone* this choice, especially persons diagnosed as mentally ill, that psychiatrists reject it. Not surprisingly, the idea of using PADs *solely* to let patients request coerced psychiatric treatment is popular among mental health professionals; by offering the patient's blessing for the psychiatrist's exercise of power, such a travesty of the PW relieves the psychiatrist of the "white man's burden."

Mental health lawyers also oppose the PW. In a 1996 law review essay, entitled "Advance directive instruments for those with mental illness," Bruce J. Winick, professor of law at the University of Miami, writes: "Some psychiatrists have responded negatively to the use of advance directive instruments in the *mental health treatment* context... However, because these may have *therapeutic value*, this negative response is unjustified."[18] Winick endorses the PW solely as an *instrument to facilitate psychiatric treatment*, thus destroying it as an instrument to enable persons to *reject the role of mental patient and avoid future psychiatric interference in their lives.*

Mental patients, Winick declares, "should be encouraged to determine in advance *how they would like to be treated* during future periods of incompetency."[19] At the same time, he opposes giving mental patients a choice between receiving and rejecting psychiatric treatment: "When the objection is to a therapeutic intervention...[there] may be reason to at least question whether the refusal of such treatment might be antitherapeutic and inconsistent with their [the patients'] welfare."[20] In other words, when the psychiatrist's decision is to treat, the patient's refusal ought to be, *ipso facto*, suspect. For Winick, this is a solution. For me, it is a problem.

In psychiatry, tradition and law sanction the use of involuntary treatment. Hence, the principal objective and use of PWs ought to be helping patients *abstain from unwanted interventions.* Winick disagrees. He writes: "The subordination of the patient's liberty interest in engaging in future mental health-care decision-making to the state's police power is no different than the state's interest in public health or safety overriding the desire of a patient suffering from infectious tuberculosis who refuses treatment."[21] Tuberculosis control laws, as we saw earlier, do not support mental health laws.[22] Winick defends his prohibiting the mental patient from divorcing the psychiatrist with this patronizing remark: "The very process of advance planning can have a number of positive therapeutic effects."[23]

Similar arguments for using PADs as instruments of psychiatric domination abound in the mental health literature. In an essay tellingly titled "Advance directives for psychiatric treatment," Robert D. Miller, a psychiatrist at the University of Colorado Health Sciences Center, writes: "If these guidelines [denying the option of rejecting treatment] are followed, then the Sirens' call of *those who would use psychiatric advance directives to frustrate, rather than further, treatment can be ignored and true patient autonomy can be supported,* not subverted."[24]

Adina Halpern and George Szmukler, an English lawyer and psychiatrist, respectively, dismiss the use of PADs as instruments of patient self-determination because, "The competent sufferer from a psychiatric disorder could reject in advance treatment which is likely to alleviate his illness, and *perhaps save his life.*"[25] However, they recommend that mental patients be permitted to elect involuntary psychiatric treatment because it "offers an ethically sound approach to reconciling *self-determination and early non-consensual treatment.*"[26]

Kay Redfield Jamison, an enthusiastic advocate of psychiatric coercion in all its forms, praises the psychiatric coercions to which she was subjected; declares the distinction between voluntary and involuntary psychiatric relations to be "misleading and arbitrary";[27] and recommends her personal version of the psychiatric will as a model for such instruments: "I drew up a clear arrangement with my psychiatrist and family that if I again become severely depressed they have the authority to approve, against my will if necessary, both electroconvulsive therapy, or ECT, an excellent treatment for certain types of severe depression, and hospitalization."[28] Jamison does not seem to recognize that if it is reasonable for her to prospectively request that she be given ECT against her will, it is just as reasonable for someone else, similarly situated, to request that she be not given ECT or any other treatment. I support Jamison's right pro-actively to reject self-responsibility and embrace psychiatric slavery *for herself.* However, she and her colleagues oppose the right of others pro-actively to accept self-responsibility and reject psychiatric slavery.

The foregoing objections to a true psychiatric will illustrate the psychiatric protectionists' conceited belief that assent to their dogmas is a mark of sanity, and their intolerant condemnation of dissent from their dogmas is a mark of insanity. *A priori*, the psychiatric testator's prospective consent to treatment is valid, but his prospective rejection of it is invalid.

Like psychiatrists, medical ethicists oppose a genuine PW because they worry that mental patients would use it to reject psychiatric treatment and kill themselves. However, they support the perverted PAD. Two Dutch medical ethicists, Guy Widdershoven and Ron Berghmans at Maastricht University, write: "By using psychiatric advance directives, it would be possible for mentally ill persons who are competent and with their disease in remission, and *who want timely intervention in case of future mental crisis, to give prior authorization to treatment* at a later time when they are incompetent... Thus the devastating consequences of recurrent psychosis could be minimized."[29]

Widdershoven and Berghmans do not recognize rejection of psychiatric care as a justifiable and valid option for the psychiatric testator. They view the status of the psychiatric slave as fixed for life: "However, even if the individual [with bipolar disorder] complies with the necessary lithium medication, a breakthrough of a manic condition cannot always be prevented." However, when such a patient is in remission, he is, according to the authors themselves, competent: "It would be required that the patient's disorder be in remission at the time the contract was made." Why, then, do they reject the seemingly self-evident proposition that a person competent to execute a valid PW requesting future psychiatric treatment is, *ipso facto*, also competent to reject such treatment? Because they see normal people and mental patients as living in different existential-moral worlds: "Voluntariness, coolness or critical reflection are possible arguments for the authority of certain wishes, but such arguments *need to be investigated and discussed. What the patient 'really' wants is the subject of joint narrative work...autonomy is not a given basis for the validity of psychiatric advance directives*, but an issue which needs constant communicative work by patient and doctor. *The psychiatric patient is not a self-sufficient individual directing her own life. She is a person in distress, and in need of care...* The danger of future psychosis is always lingering."[30]

What the *patient* wants is the subject of joint narrative work, what the *psychiatrist* wants is not. As long as the patient is a slave, and the psychiatrist is his master, the two cannot engage *jointly* in anything. Two Australian medical ethicists, Julian Savulescu and Donna Dickenson, at the University of Melbourne, also believe that giving mental patients an option to reject treatment is so wrongheaded that it ought to be impermissible: "It is difficult to establish whether a mentally ill person was competent at the time of completing an advance directive and whether the preference was the product of mental illness."[31]

It is no more difficult to establish whether a mentally ill person is competent at the time of completing an advance directive than it is to establish whether any person is competent at the time of completing an advance directive. Savulescu and Dickenson think it is because they view mentally healthy persons and mentally sick persons as radically different kinds of human beings: "Not only is a person with mental illness a risk to himself, he is also a risk to others. And preventing harm to others is a good reason to override an advance directive refusing treatment... *To encourage the use of advance directives in mental illness would be to encourage suicide.*"[32] This is an assumption stated as an assertion; even if it were true that PWs would, statistically, increase the frequency of suicide, this would not be a self-evident reason for prohibiting their use. In any case, evidence suggests that the opposite is more likely to be the case: giving people a choice to reject the mental patient role *would probably reduce homicide and suicide,* as persons often resort to these acts to avoid being placed in the role of involuntary mental patient.

As I write this, my local newspaper reports: "A man shot two deputies, killing one, before turning the gun on himself... The deputies had approached the rural home to try to serve Charles Anderson with mental commitment papers."[33] Similar stories appear frequently in the newspapers.

Implicitly, all four of the medical ethicists whose writings I cited view the role of the mental patient as a fixed status and the efficacy of treatment for mental illness as essentially nil, since it can never restore the patient to a mental state that would entitle him to exercise the same rights that non-mental patients can exercise. According to these authors, once a person is diagnosed as mentally ill, he should *never* be allowed to execute a valid psychiatric will expressing a preference for *not being treated as a mental patient.* With virtually everyone wanting to help the mental patient and hardly anyone willing to leave him alone, it is not surprising that he remains infantilized and institutionalized, a ward of the judge and the psychiatrist.

"To be Jewish," observed John Gross, long-time editor of the *Times Literary Supplement,* "was to belong to a club from which there was no resigning."[34] In the eyes of the slave owner, the same was true for Negroes: "blacks were perpetual children."[35] Even Thomas Jefferson believed that slaves were "as incapable as children of taking care of themselves."[36] In the eyes of mental health professionals, the same is true for mental patients: once considered crazy, always considered crazy.

Conclusions

The ultimate psychiatric objection against the PW lies in the belief that the person classified as a mental patient is dangerous not because of *who he is,* but because of *the illness from which he suffers*; and that, if he were freed from his illness, he would no longer be dangerous. This Jekyll-and-Hyde theory of chemicals in the brain turning "normal" people into maddened killers and self-killers is pure fantasy.

The idea of the drug as killer dates to the time of the Crusades, when it was believed that certain Shiite Muslim fanatics used hashish to transform themselves into fearless fighters. The term "assassin" is a Frankish corruption of the word "Hashishi." More recently, the power to turn men into murderers was attributed to cocaine. The idea of a drug turning men into self-killers is a modern invention, contemporaneous with the transformation of suicide from sin to sickness.[37] Drunkenness has, of course, long been blamed for violence. The Romans had a more realistic view of the effect of drugs on behavior. Their motto was, "*In vino veritas*" ("in wine the truth" or, less literally, wine loosens the tongue): the drunken person's behavior reveals his true character. Drugs do not impart any ideas or impulses to the user. Instead of blaming the drug and considering drug use an excusing condition in law, the Romans blamed the user and considered drug use an aggravating condition.

Although there is no basis for the idea that certain drugs can turn men into murderers and suicides, the belief that *psychiatric drugs* can transform perfectly normal people into killers and self-killers—like the belief that post-partum depression can transform loving mothers into the mass murderers of their own children—is simply too useful to be abandoned. The claim that untreated mental diseases cause such behaviors helps psychiatrists to impersonate real doctors (by prescribing psychiatric drugs) and puts billions into the coffers of pharmaceutical companies. The opposite claim—that psychiatric drugs cause such behavior—helps another group of psychiatrists to impersonate real doctors (as medical experts on stopping the use of psychiatric drugs) and puts billions into the pockets of trial lawyers and psychiatric experts who testify in court under oath that psychiatric drugs "cause" murder and suicide.[38]

The view that mental illness causes murder and suicide, and the view that drugs used to treat mental illness cause such behaviors, are both false. One excuses the actor from responsibility by blaming his behavior on psychiatric diseases, the other excuses him from responsibility by blaming his behavior on psychiatric treatments. Both contentions are claims serving the claimants' medical, legal, and economic interests. And both claims bolster psychiatric slavery, based equally on the insanity defense and on civil commitment. Promoting psychiatric excuses, like promoting psychiatric coercions, does not weaken psychiatric slavery, it strengthens it.

I maintain that so-called mental illness is a part of a person's identity or self, not a disease apart from him. If a person called "mental patient" is dangerous—if he assaults and kills another person, or mutilates or kills himself—it is not because of a mental disease he allegedly has, nor because of a drug he takes or does not take, but because of who he is and what he decides.

6

Jim Crow Psychiatry II:
The Patient Self-Determination Act

Many politicians of our time are in the habit of laying it down as a self-evident proposition that no people ought to be free till they are fit to use their freedom. The maxim is worthy of the fool in the old story, who resolved not to go into the water till he had learned to swim. If men are to wait for liberty till they become wise and good in slavery, they may indeed wait for ever.

—*Thomas Babington Macauley (1800-1859)[1]*

Once...insane asylums exist, there must be someone to sit in them. If not you—then I; if not I—then some third person.

—*Anton Chekhov (1860-1904)[2]*

The Psychiatric Will (PW) and the Patient Self-Determination Act (PSDA) both rest on the premise that, unless formally declared incompetent, individuals ought to be presumed competent and entitled to reject any and all meddling by health workers. Psychiatrists cannot accept this premise and endure as medical specialists. Just as the survival of slavery depended on denying the *legitimacy of the black man's unqualified humanity*, so the survival of psychiatry depends on denying the *legitimacy of the psychiatric patient's unqualified right to personhood*.

The Patient Self-Determination Act

In the nineteenth century, pathologists defined what counted as disease. Today, politicians often perform this function, especially with respect to the diseases we call "mental." The first president to assume the authority to determine what counts as a disease was John F. Kennedy. In a message to Congress in 1963, he declared: "I propose a national mental health program to assist in the inauguration

105

of a wholly new emphasis and approach to the care of the mentally ill... We need...to return mental health care to the mainstream of American medicine."[3] In 1999, at a White House Conference on Mental Health, President William J. Clinton was more specific. He asserted: "Mental illness can be accurately diagnosed, successfully treated, just as physical illness."[4] First Lady Hillary Rodham Clinton agreed: "We must...begin treating mental illness as the illness it is on a parity with other illnesses."[5] Tipper Gore, President Clinton's Mental Health Advisor, added: "One of the most widely believed and most damaging myths is that mental illness is not a physical disease. Nothing could be further from the truth."[6]

Every one of these statements is a lie. Their evident falsehood is underscored by the fact that there are no illnesses other than mental illnesses whose disease status requires validation by the White House.

The logo of the National Alliance for the Mentally Ill (NAMI), the most influential mental health lobby in the nation, proclaims: "Mental diseases are brain disorders." *Campaign Spotlight*, the organization's newsletter, explains: "In the last few years the overwhelming weight of medical research has demonstrated that mental illnesses are biologically based and that effective treatment works."[7] The equation of mind with brain, supported by a large body of neuroscience literature, justifies the drug treatment of mental illnesses and the demand for equal insurance coverage for bodily and mental illnesses.[8] Reflecting the influence of these ideas, President Clinton signed the Mental Health Parity Act of 1996 (P.L. 104-204), which became the law on January 1, 1998. NAMI hailed it as a "landmark law [that] begins the process of ending the long-held practice of providing less insurance coverage for mental illnesses, or brain disorders, than is provided for equally serious physical disorders."[9] Many states have enacted similar legislation.[10]

The assertion that medical diseases and mental diseases are on a par, that they belong in the same logical class, is false. Uremia is a literal disease. Pyromania is a metaphorical disease. We say that the patient with infectious tuberculosis *is dangerous* because he can give other people tuberculosis. However, we say that the patient with pyromania or schizophrenia *is dangerous* not because he can give other people pyromania or schizophrenia, but because we fear that he might commit arson or assault. The claim that mental illnesses are like other diseases is a fraud and doctors know it. A British study of general practitioners revealed that they "regarded psychiatric illness in themselves as a weakness. Paradoxically, they reassured patients that 'it's just another illness.'"[11] Sad to say, there is nothing paradoxical about the doctors' double-talk: they are loyal soldiers in the National Health Service; they are simply "following orders."

The medical-political debate about "parity" for mental health care is mendacious rhetoric.[12] Mental health lobbyists demand parity in insurance coverage for medical and psychiatric treatments, but oppose parity in the legal status of medical and mental patients. The truth is that the legal standings of medical patients and mental patients differ radically, and the supporters of psychiatric slavery like it that way. These differences are rationalized on the ground that medical diseases are unlikely to impair the patient's competence to assume or reject the sick role, but mental diseases are likely to do so. This justification is not based on evidence; it is based on a definition. Mental illness is that disease which impairs the patient's judgment about the benefits of involuntary psychiatric diagnosis and treatment for him.

What follows is the background against which we ought to view the Patient Self-Determination Act (PSDA) and the systematic exclusion of the mental patient from its provisions.

Enacted by Congress in 1991, the PSDA mandates that health care providers receiving Medicare and/or Medicaid payments "inform patients of their existing rights under state law to refuse treatment and prepare advance directives."[13] Specifically, it requires health care providers in hospitals, skilled nursing facilities, and other health care settings "1) to develop written policies concerning advance directives; 2) ask all new patients whether they have prepared an advance directive and include this information in the patient's chart; 3) give patients written materials regarding the facility's policies on advance directives and the patient's right (under applicable state law) to prepare such a document; and 4) educate staff and the community about advance directives."[14]

The Social Context of the PSDA

In the years after World War II, medical-technological advances, such as antibiotics, artificial methods of feeding, renal dialysis, and the ventilator, enabled physicians not only to prolong the lives of many patients, but extend their lives into states of chronic vegetative existence, often worse than death for both the patient and the family. Traditionally, the decision to employ life-saving measures was the doctor's job. The potentiality to artificially prolong life to a point that, to many, seemed not worth living, led to a popular demand for letting patients decide whether they wanted to accept or reject such medical measures. The PSDA was created to encourage people to anticipate the possibility of their being placed on life support and to prospectively request or reject such treatment. The principal objective of the PSDA was protecting patients' common law right of self-determination, defined as a constitutional "liberty interest" guaranteed by the Fourteenth Amendment. The Act invites individuals to prepare medical advance directives or living wills, offering everyone the option to *reject certain medical and surgical interventions.*

The PSDA is often discussed as if individuals were patients first, and persons second. This leads to the mistaken view that self-determination is a quality that people called "patients" lack or possess to a diminished degree, and to the conclusion that the best way to compensate for this is by politicians "giving" patients special "rights," especially the "right to die" by rejecting "life-saving treatment." This perspective is intellectually crippling. Self-determination is an aspect of self-ownership: it is the freedom to choose how to use one's body. Self-determination is an integral part of individual liberty. Limitation of self-ownership is a limitation of liberty. The similarity in the statuses of slave, prisoner, mental patient, and child lies in that the self-ownership of each is under the control of others who have legally sanctioned power over him.

How Self-Determination Is Lost

Limitation or loss of self-determination—over a specific aspect of one's life or in its entirety—can come about in three ways: by the subject's voluntary choice, by the action of another person or institution, or by the disabling effects of disease or injury. Individuals *relinquish* some of their self-determination and delegate the right to make decisions for them to spouses, dentists, doctors, and lawyers; are *deprived* of self-determination in prison, mental hospital, and the military; and *lose* some or all of their self-determination as a result of disease and disability (without relinquishing it or being deprived of it by others).

To understand the existential and legal predicament of the mental patient, we must be clear about the reasons for his loss of self-determination: we must ascertain whether his loss is voluntary, imposed by others, due to disease, or some combination of these factors, ex-emplified by behavior deliberatively provoking imprisonment or mental hospitalization. Although common knowledge, it should be emphasized that many people who love receiving the benevolent coercion of others also love to play the role of benevolent authority and coerce others. Zealots for God voluntarily submit to religious authorities, and in turn coerce and kill others in the name of God. Zealots for mental health exhibit the same behavior. Psychologist-patient Kay Redfield Jamison proudly displays her craving for be-ing subjected to psychiatric coercion and aggressively promotes the psychiatric coercion of individuals who refuse being saved by psychiatry.[15] Others, less articulate and less influential, ask to be taken care of indirectly. A homeless person cannot gain admittance to a mental hospital by knocking at the door and asking to be let in; to achieve that goal, he must act crazy and perhaps, commit a crime. The tragic story of Andrea Yates—who, in June 2001, sys-tematically drowned her five children in a bathtub—is a case in point.[16]

In 1994, after her first child was born, Yates, a trained nurse, began to have "visions." She had one child after another and, with each, her "visions" increased. In June 1999, troubled by her "visions," she "in-gested 40 to 50 pills of her father's Alzheimer's medicine." Afterward, in the hospital, she chastised herself for failing to kill herself. "'I'm a nurse. I should have known what kind of OD (overdose) to take,' she said." She was admitted to a mental hospital and treated with antipsychotic drugs. A few weeks later, she "scratched at her throat with a steak knife in search of the carotid artery. Her husband grabbed it away and took her to the hospital. 'I had a fear I would hurt somebody,' she ex-plained to a psychiatrist. 'I thought it better to end my own life and prevent it.'" She was prevented from killing herself by involuntary psychiatric hospitalization and drug treatment.

Although Yates clearly could not manage her life or take care of her children, "the Yateses stunned doctors by telling them they wanted more children. 'Patient and husband plan to have as many babies as nature will allow!' one doctor wrote. 'This will surely guarantee fur-ther psychotic depression.'" In November 2000, the couple's fifth baby was born. Yates began to deteriorate again: "She was nearly mute by the time her husband took her to the hospital in April and again in May [2001] for help. As before, the medical staff's chief concern was that Yates would harm herself, not her kids." In June, she killed all of her children. Committed to a mental hospital, her depression lifted.

Andrea Yates could not, or did not want to, admit to herself that she had assumed more obligations than she, or perhaps anyone in her situation, could have fulfilled. Although psychiatrists recognized that the Yateses' own behavior created their predicament, they treated her as if she had an acute infectious illness that could be cured with drugs. I interpret Yateses' "mental symptoms" as indirect communications, nonverbal pleas, addressed "to whom it may concern," for someone to care for her and her children. No one listened. She screamed louder and, finally, released herself from her burdens.

Consensual limitation of self-determination is an integral element of every agreement or contract, and is therefore of no further interest to us here. I shall also not consider, except in passing, loss of self-determination due to accident or disease. Present legal principles and practices governing health proxies and guardianship for medically disabled persons are adequate and appropriate remedies for this contingency. If the unconscious person is in the company of a parent, spouse, or adult child, then that person becomes, *ipso facto*, his temporary medical guardian, with the power to give or withhold consent for treatment. If no such kin is available, then the legal doctrine of *parens patriae* becomes operative: appropriate agencies of the community—acting as quasi-parents, protecting and caring for the individual as if he were a child—have the duty to care for him, until such time as he can reassume control over himself or his guardian can assume control. In what follows, I shall be concerned only with limitations to self-determination imposed on the individual against his will, by psychiatrists or by judges rubber-stamping their recommendations.

The Mental Patient and the PSDA

The patients most often deprived of the right to self-determination—specifically, of the right to refuse treatment—are mental patients. Nevertheless, in his 300-page book entitled *The Patient Self-Determination Act*, Lawrence P. Ulrich, professor of philosophy at the University of Dayton, does not mention mental patients. He states: "It [the PSDA] generally reaffirms rights that patients already possess, such as the right to refuse treatment. Unfortunately, patients have not always been aware of these rights, and *for this reason they have all too often become victims of the decisions of others.*"[17] It is no mean feat—but no doubt professionally advantageous—to ignore the plight of psychiatric patients.

Ulrich's assertion that "patients have not always been aware of these rights, and for this reason they have all too often become victims of the decisions of others" is false: the very diagnosis of mental illness negates the rights of persons so diagnosed to the benefits provided for them by the PSDA. Ulrich ignores the psychiatric will and is silent about the many ways judges, lawyers, and psychiatrists use mental health laws to deprive individuals of rights guaranteed by the Act.[18] Instead of scrutinizing how a person becomes a mental patient, Ulrich misrepresents legal and social reality by implying that the PSDA protects all patients. He writes:

> The right of patients to consent to or refuse treatments is the basis of everything to be found in this law. This is an application of the basic liberty that we all enjoy in a democratic society... [The Act] is intended to amplify autonomous decision-making by helping patients clearly understand that they can take control of their health care even to the point of refusing any or all treatments... This extension of decision-making authority beyond the onset of decisional incapacity recognizes that patients have an interest in the health care decisions that affect them even if they are no longer able to participate in them in an active and direct way.[19]

As Americans, we are supposed to have inalienable rights to life, liberty, and property. Why, then, do we need special rights when we are patients? Do we cease to be whole persons when we are patients and instead become three-fifths persons? Who deprives us of our rights when we are in the patient role? The answer is, the state—through its psychiatrist-agents. Only the state possesses legitimate authority to deprive individuals of liberty. *Psychiatrists are the only physicians who operate institutions for incarcerating persons as patients.* A private person cannot deprive another person of his rights without committing a criminal offense. People called "patients" are, first and foremost, persons. Their patient status is secondary and, as far as their legal rights are concerned, ought to be just as irrelevant as is their religious status.

Why is the self-determination of patients, especially mental patients, problematic? To understand why, we must be clear about what it means to be a patient, especially a mental patient. People often refer to individuals they regard as sick as "patients." Colloquially speaking, that is correct. However, the term "patient" has a narrower and more precise meaning: a patient is a person who occupies what sociologists call a particular "social role," in this case, the "patient role."

The patient role is a relational concept. A person is considered a patient if he consults a physician, occupies a hospital bed, or is designated a "patient" by a person or agency authorized to do so (for example, to qualify for disability compensation). A person may occupy the patient role voluntarily or involuntarily, and a person called "patient" may or may not have an illness.[20]

The term "patient," like the term "husband," refers to a role of standing-in-relation to another. Because the patient's partner is a physician, and because the physician is licensed by the state, the person-as-patient—much as the person-as-taxpayer—is an individual confronted by the only political entity legally authorized to limit his liberty: the state. That is precisely what the state, through its physician agents, does: it deprives individuals called "dangerously mentally ill" of personal liberty and responsibility, by incarcerating them in mental hospitals, declaring them unfit to stand trial, and disposing of them as not guilty by reason of insanity. Furthermore, through its physician-agents, the state deprives everyone within its borders of the liberty to purchase certain drugs without medical authorization (prescription laws).

Having deprived persons-as-patients of liberty and responsibility, the state now proposes to protect their rights to self-determination. This is something the state cannot do. If a person has the capacity to determine his own best interest, then no one else can, or ought to be able to, usurp that role. The slave owner either set his slaves free or he did not. If he manumitted them, he annulled his own right to control them; the ex-slaves' so-called best interests had nothing to do with the matter. There can be no emancipation of mental patients without annulling the psychiatrists' powers over them. And if the psychiatrist's powers are annulled, there is no need to emancipate the mental patient.

The Right to Reject (Medical) Treatment

In the West, it is a well-established medical, moral, and legal principle that an adult person's body belongs to himself and therefore medical intervention without the subject's permission constitutes assault and battery. The oldest reported case, dating back to 1767, concerns a surgeon's resetting a fractured leg without the patient's consent.[21] In 1891, in an often-cited decision, the United States Supreme Court ruled that "No right is held more sacred, or is more carefully guarded, by the common law, than the right of every individual to possession and control of his own person, free from all restraint or interference of others... The right to one's person may be said to be a right of complete immunity: to be let alone."[22] In 1928, Justice Louis D. Brandeis repeated that famous phrase, stating: "The makers of our Constitution sought to protect Americans in their beliefs, their thoughts, their emotions, and their sensations. They conferred, as against the Government, the right to be let alone—the most comprehensive of rights, and the right most valued by civilized men."[23]

It is difficult to reconcile these opinions with the practices of coercive psychiatry, unless we assume that a diagnosis of mental illness automatically removes the mental patient from the class of human beings called "persons." Even that interpretation is rendered untenable in the light of an opinion, handed down by Chief Justice (then Circuit Judge) Warren Burger in 1964, declaring that the right to be let alone attaches as well to the "irrational" decisions of "irrational" patients. In a landmark decision concerning the constitutionality of letting Jehovah's Witnesses reject life-saving blood transfusion, Burger cited Brandeis' famous admonition and then added: "Nothing in this utterance suggests that Justice Brandeis thought an individual possessed these rights only as to *sensible* beliefs, *valid* thoughts, *reasonable* emotions, or *well-founded* sensations. I suggest he intended to include a great many foolish, unreasonable, and even absurd ideas which do not conform, such as refusing medical treatment even at great risk."[24] Like the Jehovah's Witness who rejects life-saving treatment for reasons right for him but wrong for others, the mental patient rejects coercive psychiatric treatment for reasons right for him but wrong for others. If the former has a constitutional right to do so, why not also the latter? The answer, once again, lies in equating mental illness with dangerousness.

Ostensibly, the mental patient is incarcerated because he is ill and needs treatment. Actually, he is incarcerated because he is considered to be dangerous to himself and others. In a study of so-called "insanity acquittees," investigators concluded: "The public concern is clearly about dangerous persons, regardless of mental health status."[25] The history of psychiatry supports this observation.

Prior to World War II, many persons confined involuntarily in state mental hospitals suffered from paresis, a form of neurosyphilis. But having a brain disease was not the only or even the main reason why they were committed to state hospitals. Other patients with brain diseases—cerebral neoplasms, multiple sclerosis, Parkinsonism—were not committed to state hospitals. Patients with paresis were committed because, like other "insane" persons, they often exhibited disordered behaviors; patients with other diseases of the central nervous system rarely did so. In short, "mental patients" were confined against their will primarily because they misbehaved—exhibited behavior that was disturbing, threatening, or just made others uncomfortable—not because they were *sick*. This is still the case.

The fact that the PSDA is a special law to protect rights that people supposedly possess already raises the suspicion that it is unlikely to restore any rights to those now most egregiously deprived of them. Indeed, the PSDA resembles the Thirteenth Amendment. "The law," Thoreau rightly pointed out, "will never make men free; it is men who have got to make the law free."[26]

The Emancipation Proclamation, issued by President Abraham Lincoln on January 1, 1863, declared "that all persons held as slaves [within the rebellious states] are, and henceforward shall be free." The Proclamation applied only to states that had seceded from the Union, leaving slavery untouched in the loyal border states; it also exempted parts of the Confederacy that had already come under Northern control. The Emancipation Proclamation did not free a single slave.[27]

The law declared liberated slaves to be the equals of whites, but a society dominated by white-supremacist ideas separated blacks from whites and treated members of the two groups differently. Similarly, in the Patient Self-Determination Act, the law declares mental patients to be the equals of medical patients, but a society dominated by psychiatric doctrine separates the mentally ill from the mentally healthy and treats members of the two groups differently. Unlike medical patients, psychiatric patients are presumed to be incompetent, hence cannot reject psychiatric treatment or execute valid psychiatric advance directives, even after they have, ostensibly, been restored to competence.

Mental Health Disinformation

In his 1996 law review article, Winick emphasizes the differences between mental illness and medical illness and depersonalizes the commitment process. He writes: "First, the *state* may insist on psychiatric hospitalization and various forms of mental health treatment on an involuntary basis. Second, when mental illness strikes, individuals may not be able to make their own treatment decisions... [H]ow can a prudent person facing the increased possibility of an encounter with mental illness plan for the future?"[28]

The state does not hospitalize mental patients; psychiatrists do. Winick is concerned about mental patients "facing the increased possibility of an *encounter with mental illness*," and offers to allay that concern by letting them elect psychiatric enslavement. I am concerned about anyone, not just mental patients, facing the possibility of an *encounter with psychiatrists*, and want to offer them protection from that danger by letting them reject unwanted psychiatric "help."

Winick also asserts, erroneously, that "the question of the extent to which mental patients have a right to refuse treatment was first raised in the 1970's."[29] I have been raising that question since the 1950s.[30] Finally, in his book, *The Right to Refuse Mental Health Treatment*, published in 1997—six years after the PSDA was enacted into law—Winick does not even mention the Act.[31]

Elizabeth M. Gallagher, a lawyer in Seattle, Washington, also spurns the right to reject psychiatric treatment and endorses the use of PADs only as instruments for appointing proxies *to authorize psychiatric treatment*: "The case law involving the right to reject psychiatric treatment has emerged as an entirely distinct line of authority from that which has developed in the nonpsychiatric context... Whereas in the nonpsychiatric cases the state's interests are rarely regarded as sufficiently compelling to overcome the fundamental liberty interests at stake, in psychiatric cases the state's interests almost always prevail."[32] So much for the proclaimed "parity" for mental illness and the promises of the PSDA. Jim Crow psychiatry rules.

Gallagher recommends the use of PADs as a means of extending the legitimacy of psychiatric slavery: "Given the considerable deference typically accorded the state's interests in the context of civil commitment, one may legitimately question whether an advance directive would have any ascertainable impact on the course of involuntary treatment... [Still], an advance directive could always be used to *provide prospective consent to treatment*, thus obviating the need for judicial intervention."[33] In other words, Gallagher believes that persons expecting to be turned into involuntary psy-

chiatric patients are legally competent if they agree to their psychiatric self-enslavement and ought to be able to prospectively
consent to it, but if they object to psychiatric coercion, then, *ipso
facto*, they are legally incompetent and ought not to be able to reject the treatment they "need." This is not a decision by the patient to
accept treatment; it is a blessing of the psychiatrist's decision to impose it.

Misinforming the Public about Psychiatric Advance Directives

Advance directives, or so-called health proxies for medical patients, are now widely discussed not only in professional publications but also in the popular press and on many Internet sites. From
the point of view of a psychiatric abolitionist, virtually all this information is pro-psychiatric slavery propaganda, i.e., misinformation.
For example, *The Columbia Encyclopedia* (2000) offers the following definition of a health proxy:

> Legal document in which a person assigns to another person, usually called
> an agent or proxy, the authority to make medical decisions in case of inca-
> pacitation. It is, in essence, a power of attorney for health care... It differs
> from a living will, however, in that the chosen agent has the authority to deal
> with *any medical situation* that may arise, not just end-of-life situations...
> Health-care proxies go into effect when the attending physician determines
> that the patient lacks the capacity to make decisions. Prior to that time, the
> person retains all decision-making rights.[34]

Were a person who contemplates becoming a psychiatric patient
to read this item, and similar citations from other sources, he might
conclude that the problem of psychiatric coercion has been solved.
He could feel reassured that if he doesn't want to be the beneficiary
of psychiatric coercions, he could reject such intrusions on his autonomy; and that he could appoint a proxy agent who could, should
the occasion arise, reject such psychiatric services, much as a proxy
agent could reject religious burial services for an atheist. In fact, the
opposite is the case. Psychiatric power enjoys more political, medical, journalistic, and popular support than ever, and the psychiatrist's
meddling is more pervasive than ever. Americans have more to fear
from psychiatry today than in the past, in no small part because
mental health professionals and their allies are engaged in a campaign of systematically misinforming Americans about the legal,
medical, and social risks inherent in becoming a psychiatric patient.

Consider the misinformation on the web site of the New York State Attorney General's Office. It states: "Under New York's health care proxy law, any competent person can authorize another person, usually a family member, to make health care decisions, if the patient becomes unable to do so."[35]

The web site of the "Partnership for Caring" presents a similarly mendacious account: "'Advance directive' is a general term that refers to your oral and written instructions about your future medical care, in the event that you become unable to speak for yourself... Your right to accept or refuse treatment is protected by constitutional and common law... Advance directives give you a voice in decisions about your medical care when you are unconscious or too ill to communicate."[36] In practice, none of this applies to persons classified as mental patients or to medical care classified as psychiatric treatment.

Supporters of Jim Crow mental health laws are eager to give the psychiatric slave the appearance of a choice about some of the terms of his psychiatric enslavement, all the while *making sure that he cannot choose to reject the role of psychiatric slave.* The "Minnesota Advance Psychiatric Directive and Health Care Directive," prepared jointly by the Minnesota Disability Law Center and NAMI, illustrates this deliberate deception:

> The advance psychiatric directive...can be a powerful tool to help you maintain control over what happens to you in the hospital. An advance directive spells out what you want done in a time of crisis, and also enables you to choose who you want to make medical decisions for you... An advance directive may decrease the possibility of involuntary treatment. If involuntary treatment does occur, a mental health care directive may have a direct impact on the treatment you do receive, including time in the hospital, the use of medications, place of treatment and treatment plan upon release... If you are a smoker, think about how your need to smoke may be addressed. Find out what your hospital's rules are on smoking, and how your needs fit with them... Be reasonable in what you put in the directive... Also, if your directive contains obviously unreasonable instructions, you may end up raising questions about your capacity at the time you prepared your directive.[37]

Smoking is a need. Wanting to be free is not a need. In the age of psychiatry, mental patients cannot issue "obviously unreasonable instructions," because they cannot reject the authority of psychiatry. In the age of aristocracy, commoners could not have "opinions"—only aristocrats could. Famously, the Duke of Wellington "disapproved of soldiers cheering, as too nearly an expression of opinion."[38] With respect to determining who has a right to reject psychiatric treatment, psychiatrists are our aristocrats. *We can have opinions that conflict with those of priests and politicians, but we cannot have opinions that conflict with those of psychiatrists.*

- Disagreement with the priest is freedom of religion.

- Disagreement with the politician is freedom of speech.

- Disagreement with the psychiatrist is irrationality, insanity, and mental incapacity.

It is clear that *the aim of the politically correct psychiatric will is to validate the moral legitimacy of psychiatric slavery*. NAMI's version of the PW articulates this goal quite candidly. Suzanne Vogel-Scibilia—who identifies herself as "a member of NAMI Pennsylvania's Board of Directors, a practicing psychiatrist in Beaver County, and a consumer of mental health services"—explains: "NAMI Pennsylvania's Board of Directors has formed an ad hoc committee to work on promoting advance directives in the state... Psychiatric advance directives formally declare a consumer's wishes *for treatment* should he/she become incapacitated... In situations involving dangerous behavior or lethality issues, the advance directive *would not be enforced if doing so would conflict with safe medical practice.*"[39]

The psychiatric literature amply documents that mental patients are routinely denied the rights guaranteed them by the PSDA. Psychiatrists reviewed approximately 350 admissions to three psychiatric inpatient units in Virginia; they found that out of the forty-five of the patients who tried to refuse treatment, not a single one succeeded: "Psychiatrists exercised their discretion to promptly treat all patients who refused treatment... Refusers were prescribed higher doses of antipsychotic medications than were compliant patients."[40]

Disagreements between the slaveholder and the abolitionist rested on the different views each had about which human beings were entitled to liberty and which were not. Similar differences divide the psychiatric slaveholder and the psychiatric abolitionist: the former believes that psychiatric coercion is treatment and wants to protect the psychiatric patient from the dire consequences of psychiatric "neglect"; the latter believes that psychiatric coercion is punishment and wants to protect the psychiatric patient from the dire consequences of psychiatric "help." As matters stand, disagreements between these parties are settled by the psychiatric protectionist imposing his treatment on the patient, and the requirement of psychiatric slave holding, as a professional obligation, on the abolitionist psychiatrist. Psychiatric slavery, supported by custom and law, rules.

In principle, the differences between psychiatric slaveholders and psychiatric abolitionists could be resolved by means of a PW (or PAD) offering individuals the option to prospectively request or reject involuntary psychiatric interventions. In practice, this does not work. A genuine psychiatric will, legally enforced and socially accepted, would undermine the legitimacy of psychiatry. This is why mental health professionals, politicians, and the public oppose it, and civil libertarians and ex-patients ignore it.

"An invasion of armies can be resisted," wrote Victor Hugo, "but not an idea whose time has come."[41] By the same token, an idea whose time has *not* come is easily dismissed. Abolishing psychiatric slavery is such an idea.

Conclusions

Psychiatry's fundamental reason for being is to create two classes of people: persons stigmatized as mentally ill, subject to coercive psychiatric interventions, and persons not so stigmatized, not subject to such interventions.[42] Just as the mere idea of the self-determination of the slave was an insult to his master, so is the mere idea of the self-determination of the mental patient an insult to the psychiatrist. Even after he was freed, the slave remained a despised human being.[43] Even after he is declared to be recovered or in remission, the mental patient remains a feared human being, a dangerous madman.

The psychiatrist perceives the mentally ill person as so radically different from, and inferior to, himself that he views the very idea of contracting with such a person as an absurdity. Michaela Amering, an Austrian psychiatrist, observes: Mental health professionals "draw a line between themselves and patients by assuming that they will not become psychotic."[44] There is no medical disease about which physicians, *en masse,* would make such an assumption.

The hands of the psychiatrist, unlike the hands of the regular physician, are soaked in the blood of coercion. Hence, he cannot acknowledge that his doctrines and doings are insults to his victims, who experience the very existence of their oppressors as an act of delegitimization and existential violence against them. If the psychiatrist would acknowledge this, he could no longer sleep soundly at night.

The psychiatrist's hypocrisy, like the hypocrisy of the slave owner before him, is plain to all who use their eyes for seeing and their minds for thinking. Faced with a similar situation with respect to his faith, Lord Acton—a sincere, prominent Catholic—denounced the leaders of his church with these coruscating words:

> Seeing this wickedness in the present, in men apparently excellent, I cannot doubt its existence in the past. And therefore I am very unwilling, in morals, and in discussing great men, to make allowances for their time... I insist upon the greater guilt of greater men... Just as the people of the Commune seem to me altogether odious, so do the people of the Vatican... I have never found that people go wrong from ignorance, but from want of consciousness. Even the ignorant are ignorant because they wish to be—ignorant in bad faith.[45]

I hold psychiatrists responsible for their crimes against humanity, their willful ignorance fueled by their bad faith.

7

Expanding Psychiatric Slavery:
Outpatient Commitment

The negro slaves of the South are...the freest people in the world... They
enjoy liberty, because they are oppressed neither by care or labor.
                              —*George Fitzhugh (1806-1881)[1]*

When modern absolutism arose, it laid claim to every thing on behalf of
the sovereign power. Commerce, industry, literature, religion were all
declared to be matters of State, and were appropriated and controlled
accordingly.
                              —*Lord Acton (1834-1902)[2]*

For the better part of three hundred years, it was accepted legal
practice and psychiatric dogma that mad-doctors, alienists, and psychiatrists had the power as well as the duty to forcibly restrain and
"treat" persons called "certifiable lunatics." Either a person was committable, in which case psychiatrists were, in effect, his medical custo-
dians and guardians, or he was not committable, in which case he
was safe from psychiatric coercion.

For centuries, the walls of the madhouse formed the borders of
the psychiatric slave states. Inside the walls, the psychiatrists were
the masters, and the patients the slaves. Outside the walls lay the
free psychiatric states. Persons living in that zone enjoyed liberty
from psychiatry. This is no longer true. The borders of the madhouse now extend to the outermost geographic and legal limits of
the American empire. The psychiatrist's coercion of the patient is
defined as care and he is empowered to "treat" potentially anyone,
in a "hospital without walls."[3]

The forcible deinstitutionalization of mental patients and the forcible administration of antipsychotic drugs to them, both inside and

outside mental hospitals, have radically transformed the psychiatric landscape. Hundreds of thousands of individuals diagnosed as mentally ill have been expelled from mental institutions and now live "in the community." However, the law treats such persons very differently than it treats medical patients discharged from medical hospitals. Patients discharged from mental hospitals remain under indefinite psychiatric supervision, subject to psychiatric "recall" at a moment's notice; are expected to take psychiatric drugs, intended to render them passive and compliant; are often housed in government-supported, quasi-psychiatric institutions, such as half-way houses; and are supported by government disability checks, often administered for them by others. In effect, they are on indefinite psychiatric probation.

Involuntary Outpatient Commitment

Like insulin shock, metrazol shock, electric shock, and lobotomy, antipsychotic drugs are psychiatric inventions devised and used to subdue and pacify troublesome individuals. Most patients do not like to be subjected to these interventions. That is why, for the most part, such "treatments" have been and continue to be imposed by force. These "therapies" benefit psychiatrists, the drug and device manufacturers, the patient's relatives, and society—not the patients.

These inconvenient facts pose a big problem for mental health professionals given to celebrating the therapeutic triumphs of their policy of drugs and deinstitutionalization. Because patients with mental illnesses such as schizophrenia cannot be relied on to medicate themselves the way patients with physical illnesses such as diabetes can, psychiatrists have successfully sought to extend therapeutic coercion from inside the insane asylum to the outside world. The result is a society in which the practices of psychiatric slavery reach into every nook and cranny of the community. Instead of the nation being psychiatrically half-slave and half-free, *it is now psychiatrically all-slave*.

The cure wrought by drugs-and-deinstitutionalization, like the cures produced by previous psychiatric "miracles," proved to be worse than the disease. Freed from the shackles of inpatient psychiatric slavery, the ex-slaves stopped taking the drugs that supposedly made their liberation possible and began to upset people "in the community." E. Fuller Torrey puts it this way: "A million Americans who suffer from schizophrenia or manic-depressive illness are homeless, and thousands commit violent crimes...because they don't take the drugs that could relieve their delusions and hallucinations."[4] In the 1970s, to remedy the problems created by deinstitutionalization and noncompliance with outpatient (drug) treatment, psychiatrists and lawyers extended the commitment process from inpatients to outpatients: thus was "outpatient commitment" (OC) conceived and brought into the world. By 1999, forty states and the District of Columbia had commitment statutes "permitting mandatory outpatient treatment."[5] In the antebellum South, there were two kinds of chattel slaves: plantation slaves in the field, and domestic slaves in the home. In postbellum America, there are two kinds of psychiatric slaves: inpatient psychiatric slaves in mental hospitals, and outpatient psychiatric slaves in the community.

Outpatient Commitment Defined

Inpatient commitment, like outpatient commitment, is a legal-psychiatric mechanism for forcing certain people to submit to certain psychiatric interventions against their will.

The APA's "Resource Document on Mandatory Outpatient Treatment" (1999) defines OC as follows: "Mandatory outpatient treatment refers to court-ordered outpatient treatment for patients who suffer from severe mental illness and who are unlikely to be compliant with such treatment without a court order. Mandatory outpatient treatment is a *preventive treatment* for those who do not presently meet criteria for inpatient commitment."[6]

OC laws are generally believed to authorize the forcible treatment of certain mental patients; yet, it is not clear whether they actually authorize such force or are simply used as if they do authorize it. The APA's "Resource Document" is unclear about this point: "Although most statutes and much of the literature use the term outpatient commitment, many psychiatrists prefer other phrases, such as 'mandatory outpatient treatment' or 'assisted outpatient treatment' to refer to this practice. The phrase 'outpatient commitment' implies a much more coercive approach than is envisioned by proponents of judicial treatment orders or directives."[7]

E. Fuller Torrey and Robert J. Kaplan, the latter an official of the Virginia chapter of NAMI, offer a more straightforward definition: "Outpatient commitment is a form of civil commitment in which the court orders an individual to comply with a specific outpatient treatment program. The legal authority for outpatient commitment is the state's *parens patriae* power, which provides for protection of disabled individuals, and its police power, which involves protection of others."[8]

As a practical matter, the procedure for outpatient commitment, like the procedure for inpatient commitment, is a charade. "Once a petition [for OC] has been presented," reports Tracy L. Benford, a forensic psychiatrist at Bellevue Hospital Center in New York, "very few cases have been rejected by the courts...the courts almost always accept the recommendations contained in the testimony of psychiatrists."[9] This is not because the defendant-patients do not protest against the deprivation of liberty their adversaries seek to impose on them. It is because most patients are poor, cannot secure the services of a psychiatrist to testify on their own behalf, or, if they can, the judge dismisses the patient's psychiatrist's unwelcome opinion as the unscientific, unprofessional plea of a charlatan.

How do mental health professionals implement the goal of OC? They do so by means of "community treatment programs...[that] attempt to engage reluctant patients in treatment via a process of compassionate interest and a willingness to participate in routine activities, such as helping someone obtain food, housing, or disability benefits. The teams bring medication to patients' homes."[10] In other words, the treatment teams try to bribe the patients to do the psychiatrists' bidding. If that fails, the patients can be recommitted and treated against their will in the hospital. Some thirty years ago I suggested that "what we call 'schizophrenia' is often a cry for housing."[11] Psychiatrists dismissed that characterization as a denial of the reality of schizophrenia as a disease. Now they are proud of treating schizophrenia by providing housing for patients.[12]

The question remains: How do psychiatrists get psychiatric drugs into their patients' bodies? According to psychologist Randy Borum and his colleagues, "although [the mandated treatment] order does direct the respondent [patient] to comply with prescribed treatment, *it does not permit the requirement to be forcibly enforced.* However, *respondents may have believed that they can be forced to comply.*"[13] Mental health professionals encourage that false belief. In any case, psychiatric outpatients who refuse to take prescribed drugs can always be committed and then forcibly drugged.

Does Outpatient Commitment Work?

In a word, the answer is no.[14] However, this is unimportant. What is important is that OC laws, like drug laws and gun laws, create the delusion that "the problem" is being dealt with, and is being dealt with scientifically, humanely, and effectively. In short, the laws make politicians and the public feel good. The authorities declare victory and the public basks in collective self-flattery.

In 2001, the prestigious Rand Corporation released its research report, titled "The Effectiveness of Involuntary Outpatient Treatment," together with a shorter, summarizing document, titled "Does involuntary outpatient treatment work?"[15] The researchers emphasize that they conducted (what they considered) an "empirical study" of "involuntary treatment [which] has been the most consistently debated issue in mental health law for the last thirty years. The goals of involuntary treatment have not changed radically over time: insuring public safety, guaranteeing access to treatment for those who need it, and insuring that treatment is provided in the least restrictive environment consistent with the needs of the individual."[16] Only attaining the first goal, insuring public safety, is empirically verifiable. The other goals are parts of the time-honored psychiatric rhetoric aimed at disguising the true goal of psychiatric coercion, making troublesome persons less troublesome.[17]

The Rand researchers' study confirms this view. They write: "In the last decade, however, the focus of involuntary treatment has changed as states have amended or interpreted their existing involuntary commitment statutes to allow for involuntary outpatient treatment and other *mechanisms designed to extend the state's supervisory control over mentally ill persons into the community*."[18] How did the Rand researchers overcome the obstacle of an absence of biological markers for mental illness? How do they determine whether a patient recovers, remains the same, or relapses? By using *social markers* for assessing patient status: they infer the severity of mental illness and the effectiveness of involuntary psychiatric treatment from how much trouble the patient causes others. Unsurprisingly, their conclusions are vacuous: "There is no evidence that a court order is necessary to achieve compliance and good outcomes, or that a court order, in and of itself, has any independent effect on outcomes."[19]

Is it morally justifiable to compel competent adults, living in the community, to ingest mind-altering drugs? Is it ethical to "study" such an immoral social policy? The Rand researchers neither ask nor answer such questions. Instead, they assume the posture of disinterested investigators. "Our task," they write, "is to set out the evidence so the debate can be an informed one. It is up to others to advocate, armed with an understanding of what is known from empirical work and what remains to be known."[20] This will not do. Americans in the antebellum South "studied" the involuntary cultivation of cotton and concluded that it was a boon for the economy as well as for the slaves. The Germans under Nazism "studied" the involuntary manufacture of armaments and concluded that it was economically effective and liberating for the laborers (*Arbeit macht frei. [Work makes you free.]*). In retrospect, we condemn such studies as immoral, because the mode of production studied was immoral. Notwithstanding the Rand researchers' disclaimers, their study is also immoral, because the mode of medical intervention they studied was itself immoral. If a medical intervention is imposed on a competent individual against his will, it is assault, not treatment. If behavior is not an illness, then the use of force to change it ought to be called "assault," not "treatment."

Regardless of the effectiveness of OC, psychiatrists enthusiastically support it. Torrey writes: "People will not accept medication if they don't think they're sick. That's why people with severe mental illness must be treated involuntarily."[21] Torrey implies that patients who reject being drugged are, *ipso facto,* incompetent to make rational decisions about how they want doctors to treat them. This inference is unjustified. Furthermore, even if that were true, it would not justify the physician's acting as the patient's guardian; instead, it would require that a court appoint a guardian for the patient. It would be this guardian's duty to accept or reject medical care for the patient.

Torrey loves the media and his affection is reciprocated. A reporter for the *Washington Post* repeats his mantra as if it were medical science: "Torrey has emerged as America's most prominent spokesman for the idea that the government should compel the insane to take the anti-psychotic drugs that can relieve their illness. A million Americans who suffer from schizophrenia or manic-depressive illness are homeless, and thousands commit violent crimes, Torrey says, because they don't take the drugs that could relieve their delusions and hallucinations."[22] Sally Satel agrees: "About half of all schizophrenics have no insight into their own condition and no understanding of why they need medication. As for free will, *the freedom to be psychotic is no freedom at all.*"[23]

Mental health professionals and lawmakers assume that inpatient commitment and outpatient commitment are effective and legitimate policies for insuring that severely ill mental patients receive treatment. However, there is no evidence to support this assumption, and it is questionable whether it is morally justifiable to use compulsion for such a purpose. I have long maintained that it is not. George Hoyer, professor of community medicine at the University of Tromse, in Norway, agrees. He writes:

> Most of the arguments supporting civil commitment can be questioned... Seriously mentally disordered patients neither lack insight, nor is their competency impaired to the degree previously believed. The superior outcome of coerced treatment has not been demonstrated... The lack of scientifically sound studies concerning the outcome of civil commitment and coercive treatment leaves mental health professionals in a difficult situation when civil commitment is considered... [T]here seems to be a general agreement that civil commitment of patients who are dangerous to themselves or others should be the responsibility of the mental health care system, while civil commitment for treatment purposes is more controversial and hard to justify.[24]

Hoyer's statement that "civil commitment for treatment purposes is...hard to justify" ought to be of particular interest to American jurists and psychiatrists who love to bask in the glory of Americans' "right" to *involuntary psychiatric treatment*, allegedly guaranteed by the Constitution. In the celebrated *Donaldson* case, a Florida trial court in 1974 ruled that "The purpose of involuntary mental hospitalization is treatment."[25] The ruling was upheld by the Fifth Circuit Court of Appeals, which held "that the Fourteenth Amendment guarantees involuntarily civilly committed mental patients a right to treatment."[26]

Judicial discoveries about Constitutional guarantees of involuntary psychiatric treatment, and the psychiatric fabrications on which they are based, are simply noise and fury, signifying only the unassailable legal legitimacy of psychiatric slavery. It is the security of that legitimacy that explains why, after successfully implementing one new "reform" after another, psychiatrists continue to make ever new demands for more rights to oppress patients, and more funds with which to do it. In the aftermath of the deinstitutionalization that psychiatrists themselves demanded and executed, they and their acolytes began to lament the "criminalizing of mental illness" and the "lack of mental health services," especially for children.[27] Surgeon

General David Satcher asserts: "Too often, children who are not iden-tified as having mental health problems and who do not receive ser-vices end up in jail."[28] Healer General Jesse Jackson declares: "You must fight tooth and nail against those who would imprison people who have mental illnesses... We must be sane. We must be sane. We must fight for sanity... We are a God-blessed nation... You, as good psychologists...help us find all the lost sheep."[29]

Persons with psychiatric diagnoses are in prisons not because they are sick, but because they are lawbreakers. Persons with psychiatric diagnoses who are forcibly drugged are not lost sheep; they are per-sons entitled to liberty and ought to be held responsible for their actions.

Outpatient Commitment: Cui Bono?

For centuries, psychiatrists insisted that the intended and actual beneficiaries of involuntarily hospitalized mental patients were the coerced patients, not their families and society. Now, they insist that the intended and actual beneficiaries of involuntary outpa-tient commitment are the coerced patients, not their families and society.

In 2000, New York State enacted its version of an outpatient com-mitment law, named Kendra's Law, after Kendra Webdale, a young woman pushed to her death under a subway train by a "schizo-phrenic" patient released from a mental hospital. This law, a psy-chiatrist states, "was originally going to be named the 'Assisted Out-patient Treatment Act,' to denote that its intent was to help patients in dire need of treatment."[30] The psychiatrist describing the develop-ment of the law does not cite the views of any patients allegedly benefited by the legally mandated treatment. Instead, she cites the views of a man whose schizophrenic son refused treatment and was forcibly medicated. Kendra's law, said the father, "certainly helped my son."

In no other area of medicine is a single anecdote permitted to be used to support a theory, much less a treatment or public health policy. In other areas of medical decision making, statistical out-comes of results based on studies of groups of similar cases are used to reach conclusions. Because one so-called schizophrenic kills a woman does not mean that the risk of being killed by a person with a psychiatric diagnosis is greater than the risk of being killed by someone in the general population without such a diagnosis. However, because such persons have been subjected, often over long periods, to systematic psychiatric humiliation and coercion, they finally may channel their anger and frustration randomly against others. That completes the circle: the psychiatrist is proved right.

For nearly half a century, from all over the world, I have been receiving a steady stream of letters from individuals who feel they have been the victims of psychiatric coercion. The following excerpt from such a letter presents a patient's perspective on outpatient commitment.

March 24, 2001

Dear Dr. Szasz,...Not too long ago I told my psychologist/social worker at XYZ Hospital [in a metropolitan area] that I did not want to come to the therapy sessions or see the psychiatrist any more. Nonetheless, the psychologist kept sending letters to my home and even telephoned my mom when I had been away from home. At the time, my mom told him that she did not know where I was. The psychologist then notified the police. When I returned home after several days, I "found" ten police officers surrounding me in my home, telling me that I had to go to XYZ Hospital Psychiatric Emergency. The police officers had opened my door without any kind of "order" or warrant. I then told them that they had no right to force me to go to the ER. The police then grabbed me and hit me with an electric stun gun... When the police brought me to the Emergency Room the psychiatrist ordered an injection when I told him that I did not want to take pills... The doctor told me that I had to go to the hospital treatment program. I did not have much of a choice. I "agreed" to go to the treatment program out of fear. Currently, I am in the hospital treatment program and afraid to quit because the police might be sent to my home again... My mom insists that I see a psychiatrist. She also wants me to continue with the program... Dr. Szasz, I feel helpless because my rights have been taken away...

This man was living in his mother's home. Evidently, she found it easier to live with him when he was being drugged by psychiatrists. The vignette illustrates that OC "works": It helps the patient's mother tolerate living with her grown, unemployed son.

Outpatient Commitment and the "Criminalizing of Mental Illness"

The core element of psychiatric slavery, the coercive control of the mental patient by the psychiatrist, has not changed since the seventeenth century. What has changed and changes continuously, is the psychiatrist's method of coercion, the scope of his powers, and the legal and social justifications for his use of force. These transformations reflect changing fashions in legal reasoning, psychiatric treatment, and popular opinion about mental illness and psychiatry.

In the 1950s, psychiatrists rarely used phrases such as "coercive treatment" or "involuntary mental hospitalization." Instead, they simply referred to mental patients being "admitted" to hospitals and receiving "treatment." Today, psychiatrists do not shy away from using the term "coercion" and face objections both from ex-patients ("psychiatric survivors" making up the absurdly misnamed "mental health consumer movement") and soi-disant psychiatric critics. However, these opponents make it easy for the psychiatric slaveholders: they are fervent believers in mental illness, the insanity defense, and even involuntary mental hospitalization.[31] For example, Phyllis Chesler, a prominent feminist psychologist, proudly affirms her belief in mental illness and the legitimacy of involuntary mental hospitalization for the "truly" mentally ill. In the foreword to a volume on the "false commitment" of sane women to insane asylums, she writes: "Do these accounts of institutional brutality and torture mean that mental illness does not exist...? Not at all. What these accounts document is that many women in the asylum were not insane..."[32] Implicitly, the other women in the asylum were insane. Chesler offers no definition of insanity and gives no hint about how we might distinguish the sane from the insane.

The psychiatric survivors' criticisms are compromised by their co-optation by the mental health movement and dependence on disability payments for mental illness. Some former mental patients even join forces with coercive psychiatrists and sing the praises of involuntary treatment. Others complain about the psychiatric services offered by the present system and demand services of their own design. All of them seem to believe that they are entitled to social security disability payments for suffering from diseases whose existence they deny.

Confronted with this new social scene, and armed with what they believe are psychiatric wonder drugs, psychiatrists have revised their rank ordering of justifications for psychiatric oppression. Now, they justify coercion primarily in order to "liberate the patient from the shackles of his illness." Protecting the public from dangerous mental patients comes next. Finally, they justify therapeutic coercion as a way to avoid "criminalizing mental illness," a phrase used to mask the psychiatric control of persons who break the law but whose lawlessness psychiatrists attribute to mental illness.

Laurie Flynn, Executive Director of NAMI, explains: "[M]ore than a quarter of a million people with schizophrenia, bipolar disorder, and other severe mental illnesses languish in the nation's prisons and jails—nearly six times the number in hospitals... Most have committed minor, non-violent offenses *caused by the symptoms of untreated illness.*"[33] If Flynn believes that symptoms cause, or can cause, crimes, then she does not know the meaning of the word "symptom." If she means that untreated mental illness causes crime, then she asserts a psychiatric cliché for which, in the absence of organic markers for mental illness, there can be no evidence.

Testifying before a hearing of the House Judiciary Subcommittee on Crime in 2000, Dr. Bernard S. Arons, Director of the Center for Mental Health Services in the U.S. Department of Health and Human Services, stated: "[B]oth the criminal justice system and mental health care system have a common problem; people with mental illness increasingly becoming involved in the criminal justice system, resulting in an increased burden on the criminal justice system and less effective treatment for the individuals involved."[34]

In addition to justifying OC as preventing unjust punishment of the mentally ill and the clogging of the prison system, psychiatrists have taken to justifying it as a method for preventing homelessness. Steven S. Sharfstein—president and medical director at the Sheppard Pratt Health System, a not-for-profit behavioral health care system in Baltimore, and clinical professor of psychiatry at the University of Maryland—relates: "Recently, half the patients on the dual-diagnosis unit at Sheppard Pratt were homeless... The revolving door of hospitalization for mental illness has already become a huge turnstile, disgorging mental patients onto the streets or into jails."[35] Psychiatrists insist that mental illnesses are medical diseases. However, discharging medical patients from medical hospitals does not result in creating hordes of homeless persons, many of whom commit criminal offenses.

In the end, Sharfstein admits that "Fear of violence has traditionally justified the concept of involuntary hospitalization... Patients are now admitted not simply because they are ill, but because they are dangerous. The criteria [sic] for retention within the hospital is continued *risk, and nothing more.*"[36] And John R. Lion, professor of psychiatry at the University of Maryland, concedes that psychiatry is fake medicine. He writes: "Psychiatry has tried so hard to fashion itself as a medical discipline that it has shot itself in the foot. Recovery from mental illness does not obey the laws of physical illness... Society doesn't want to see mental patients, whether they reside within hospitals or at half-way houses. It doesn't want to see them, period. As for hospitals, I think we will need them more and more."[37] Lion is right. *We* will need (mental) hospitals more and more, because such hospitals serve *our* interests. However, mental patients do not need mental hospitals; *they* need asylums—places of refuge where they would be *protected from coercion* by persecutors posing as protectors.[38]

Deinstitutionalization: Solution or Problem?

In the 1960s and 1970s, psychiatrists, allied with politicians, promoted deinstitutionalization as scientific progress and psychiatric reform, and declared it a great success, a "new era in psychiatry."[39] A decade later, the same "experts" declared that deinstitutionalization was a tragic failure. Why was it a failure? The answer depended on whether psychiatrists were looking for a culprit to blame it on, or were looking to the federal government for more money for psychiatric services "denied" to deinstitutionalized patients.

"From the Man Who Brought You Deinstitutionalization" was the title that John Monahan, a psychologist and professor of law at the University of Virginia, gave to his review of my book *Insanity: The Idea and Its Consequences*. In addition to blaming, or crediting, me for single-handedly bringing about the deinstitutionalization of mental patients not only in the United States but also in the United Kingdom and several European countries, he dismissed my objections to psychiatric slavery with this summary: "The crux of Szasz's philosophic position is that psychiatric and psychological practice should be based not on what he derisively refers to as 'coercive paternalism,' but on the more lofty 'principle of free contract.' The problem he seems unable to recognize is that this ideological preference is fundamentally at odds with the societal preferences that have shaped our public policy for the past 50 years."[40] Monahan willfully misinterprets my criticism of the trend he describes, which, some forty years ago I dubbed the Therapeutic State, with an inability to recognize it.[41]

Refusing to acknowledge the distinction between voluntary and involuntary human relations, Monahan states: "Szaszian has become an adjective that connotes lack of subtlety in thought and an excess of polemics in argument."[42] I maintain that there can be no such thing as a nonpolemical argument about a social policy that entails depriving innocent persons of liberty.

The idea that deinstitutionalization was my fault has, despite its absurdity, become popular. Psychiatrist Mary D. Bublis declares: "If ever there was anyone who almost single-handedly was responsible for the current mess involving the homeless mentally ill, Szasz—with his 'urgings' to 'empty the state hospitals' back in the 60's and 70's—could be that person."[43] Rael Jean Isaacs and Virginia C. Armat, authors of *Madness in the Streets*, write: "The mental health bar has substantially realized the vision of Thomas Szasz... The counterculture denied the very existence of mental illness...[as] formulated in the prolific writings of psychiatrist Thomas Szasz... The antipsychiatry movement that shut the state hospitals created an inhumane world on the streets."[44] According to Isaacs and Armat, the cruel consequences of deinstitutionalization represent "the triumph of Thomas Szasz."[45] According to Thomas G. Gutheil, "He [Szasz] was popular as a sixties kind of guy, an anti-establishment rebel... The damage he has done to the care of the mentally ill has not been carefully assessed and cannot be overestimated."[46]

Psychiatrists blame me for deinstitutionalization only when it suits their purposes. Sharfstein was closer to telling the real reason for deinstitutionalization when, testifying before a House Subcommittee hearing in 2000, he stated: "The most significant cause of deinstitutionalization was economics... The economic opportunity to shift costs from state to the federal government [has] resulted in fewer than 60,000 patients hospitalized today in public settings, down from over 500,000 forty years ago.... State hospitals have closed and continue to close without adequate resources to care for these patients in community based settings."[47] Sharfstein then re-interpreted the triumph of drugs and deinstitutionalization as the tragedy of "criminalizing the mentally ill":

> Our mission today differs little from when we were founded 150 years ago... I will describe to you the scope of criminalization of the mentally ill which I believe is a public health tragedy... With 3,500 and 2,800 mentally ill inmates respectively, the Los Angeles County jail and New York Riker's Island jail are currently the two largest psychiatric inpatient treatment facilities in the country... The warehousing of the mentally ill in jails and prisons is an unacceptable throwback to the deplorable conditions in the 19th century which prompted Dorothea Dix and the Quakers...to develop asylum care... In many if not most areas across the country, mentally ill individuals who have committed non-violent property crimes or are arrested for vagrancy have found their way inappropriately into jails or prisons.[48]

Sharfstein does not acknowledge that there never was such a thing as true deinstitutionalization. Patients in mental hospitals were never simply discharged. Instead, most of them were transinstitutionalized: elderly patients were rehoused in nursing homes; most non-elderly patients were relocated in half-way houses and other parapsychiatric establishments; many were, indeed, "discharged to the streets," engaged in criminal behavior, and ended up in prisons. It is absurd to call this process "criminalizing" mental patients, an interpretation that implies treating innocent individuals as if they were criminals.

Sharfstein's remedy for criminalizing the mentally ill is "court ordered treatment... Individuals who experience the tragedy of mental illness must be treated and not punished... The problem is we need more money, and we have to turn to the government to get it. If we [psychiatrists] don't get it, the problems will grow."[49] Sadly, the opposite is the case. The more money the government pumps into the psychiatric system, the worse the system becomes, for patient and physician alike. The remedy lies in facing the facts, creating non-coercive alternatives for the needs of the so-called homeless mentally ill, or leaving them alone. One such alternative would be a truly voluntary psychiatric system for those who want to take advantage of what it might offer. Another alternative would be a modern system of asylums—not for mental patients, but for anyone who seeks refuge, for whatever reason. In return for protecting the asylum-seeker from the demands of the "real" world, and letting him be idle, he would have to be willing to respect the rights of others by eschewing lawlessness, or suffer the penalties of the criminal justice system for his behavior.

The Lost World of the Asylum

Throughout this book, I have distinguished between the two traditional functions of psychiatry: coercing and caring. At present, psychiatry's coercive functions are growing and enjoying a high degree of legitimacy and popularity, while its caring functions are rapidly diminishing and are on the verge of disappearing.

By escalating the coercive functions of psychiatry, we engage in an unwinnable war against human nature itself. We ought to reverse course, abolish psychiatric slavery, and re-embrace psychiatry's caring and custodial functions, epitomized by the term "asylum." Long ago, I suggested that what we need are not hospitals where people are diagnosed with, and treated for, nonexistent diseases, but orphanages for unwanted adults, where such individuals could seek protection from those who might prey on them.[50] This goal could be best achieved in and by an institutional system that is philosophically and financially separate from the state, medicine, psychiatry, and the mental health industry. To be effective, such an asylum would have to grow out of the moral and social milieu of the community whose unhappy members would compose its clientele, and whose politicians and philanthropists would have to support it with the appropriate legislation and the necessary funds.

I have no intention of painting a rosy picture of the old state mental hospitals. However, prior to World War II, for some inmates, some of these hospitals fulfilled a useful function as an asylum. Since then, state mental hospitals—and private mental hospitals as well—have been *completely transformed, from asylums into hospitals, or, more precisely, pseudo-hospitals.* Our society provides no place of refuge for the individual who wants to escape from the world. Instead of offering asylum, the modern mental hospital offers only coercions called "treatments," intended to force the patient back into a society in which he cannot, or does not want to, find a place for himself.[51] Psychiatrists, and the public, refuse to acknowledge that there are many persons who—temporarily or indefinitely, and without any medically identifiable reason for disability—simply cannot, or will not, deal with the daily responsibilities of living.

During much of the nineteenth century, psychiatrists, patients, and the public accepted that insanity was incurable. This therapeutic nihilism, recognizing a reality we deny, was, paradoxically, liberating, for both patient and psychiatrist. If the patient was in the mental hospital because of dementia due to neurosyphilis or stroke or trauma, his condition was seen as a medical problem for which there was no remedy; he was cared for and was otherwise unmolested by medical personnel. If the patient was in the hospital because he was unable to cope with his life, his condition was seen as a psychiatric problem—a categorization whose exact meaning remained conveniently unclear. For this ailment, too, there was no remedy; the patient was given room and board, often a job in the institution, and sometimes— if he had talent and the luck of having a psychiatrist who recognized it and respected him—opportunity to cultivate it. In any case, the asylum doctor did not pressure the inmate to submit to treatment or leave the institution. This is why many mental patients spent their

entire lives in mental hospitals, sometimes performed socially useful services, and frequently outlived their psychiatrists.

The Unbearable Burden of Being

The contemporary reader—unless he happens to be a student of
psychiatric history—is unaware of the vast cultural, legal, and medical gap that separates the psychiatric scene before World War II, and
especially before World War I, from the contemporary psychiatric
scene. Instead of describing that world, I shall try to recreate it by
brief sketches of three famous madmen: Vincent van Gogh (1853-
1890), the Dutch painter; Dr. William Chester Minor (1834-1920),
one of the main contributors to the *Oxford English Dictionary*; and
Robert Walser (1878-1956), a Swiss poet and novelist.

Vincent van Gogh

Van Gogh's life was brutish and short. Except for his dependence
on, and closeness to, his older brother, Theo, he was friendless, pen-
niless, homeless, and generally unwanted. He spent the last third of
his short life in and out of mental hospitals.

About eighteen months before he fatally shot himself in Arles, he
famously cut off one of his ears and presented it to a prostitute he
frequented. A newspaper reported: "On Sunday last, at 11:30 p.m.,
one Vincent Vangogh [sic], a painter, born in Holland, arrived at
House of Tolerance [brothel] No. 1, asked for one Rachel, and handed
her his ear, saying 'Keep this and treasure it.' Then he disappeared.
Informed of this action, which could only be that of a poor lunatic,
the police went to the man's address the next morning and found
him lying in bed and giving almost no sign of life. The unfortunate
was admitted to hospital as an emergency case."[52]

Van Gogh himself believed that he belonged in a madhouse. In
his letters to Theo he wrote:

- I am thinking of frankly accepting my role of a madman, the way
  Degas acted the part of a notary.[53]

- Here, except for liberty, I am not too badly off.[54]

- As far as I can judge, I am not properly speaking a madman... All I
  would ask would be that people do not meddle with me when I am

busy painting, or eating, or sleeping, or taking a turn at the brothel, since I haven't a wife.[55]

• Above all, do not imagine that I am unhappy... I want you to consider this going into an asylum as a pure formality... Where I have to follow a rule, as here in the hospital, I feel at peace... I shall always be cracked.[56]

Vincent Van Gogh remained lucid to the end. In May 1890, two months before killing himself, he wrote to Theo: "I have seen Dr. Gachet, who gives me the impression of being rather eccentric, but his experience as a doctor must keep him balanced enough to combat the nervous trouble from which he certainly seems to be suffering at least as seriously as I."[57] One hundred years later, van Gogh's "Portrait of Dr. Gachet" sold for $82.5 million, then the highest price ever paid for a painting.

What was "wrong" with van Gogh? Let us see briefly how van Gogh saw himself and how others saw him.

Van Gogh saw himself as an over-sensitive person, poorly equipped to cope with life. To his brother, Theo, who supported him throughout most of his life, he wrote: "You know well enough how little fit I am to cope either with dealers or with amateurs, and how contrary it is to my nature... Money plays a brutal part in society... I have a horror of success... *All I ask in painting is a way of escaping from life*... Work is the only remedy; if that does not help, one breaks down."[58]

A librarian at the Municipal Library in Arles stated: "Vincent lives in my memory, as an extremely timid man, a child. I was not interested in him because of his art... To me he was an unhappy man, who suffered much."[59]

Psychiatrists say that van Gogh had schizophrenia. For journalists and the public, he is the very model of the mad genius. By viewing van Gogh and so-called schizophrenics as mentally ill, we not only deny them the last vestiges of dignity and personhood, we also deny ourselves the chance to understand them and to better understand the human condition.

William Chester Minor, M.D.

William Chester Minor, the scion of old American aristocracy, was born in Ceylon—now Sri Lanka—of missionary parents. After his breakdown, he attributed his troubles to seeing the native girls cavorting naked on the beach: they "had unknowingly set him on the spiral path to his eventual insatiable lust, to his incurable madness, and to his final perdition."[60] Raised by puritanical missionaries, Minor grew up to be an adult obsessed with sex. He was anxious to reassure his doctors that, despite "his fantasies over the young Indian girls, he 'never gratified himself in an unnatural way.'"[61] He regularly frequented houses of prostitution, and felt hugely guilty for doing so. I assume that, his protestations notwithstanding, he engaged in "self-abuse" and felt hugely guilty for that practice as well. His subsequent penile self-amputation supports this hypothesis.

When Minor was three, he lost his mother to tuberculosis. His father then married the daughter of an American missionary family in Bangkok. At fourteen, Minor returned to New Haven, to live with his uncle and attend Yale University. After finishing college, he went to Yale medical school, specialized in surgery, and signed on as a medical officer with the Union Army. He served honorably in the Civil War but was deeply scarred by the experience, especially by having had to brand Irish deserters. Guilt over this abuse of his medical oath haunted him for the rest of his life and formed the principal theme of his paranoid delusion.

After the war ended, Minor reenlisted, and soon his behavior began to deteriorate. His superiors dealt with his increasing ineffectiveness by assigning him to less responsible positions and finally recommended that he be sent to the Government Hospital for the Insane in Washington, D.C. A physician noted: "Doctor Minor has expressed willingness to go to the Asylum."[62] The initial diagnosis, made by an Army physician in 1868, was "monomania." Two years later, he was discharged from the hospital and was given an honorable medical discharge from the Army, with full pay for the rest of his life and the right to use the title, "US Army, Ret'd."

Minor was then thirty-four years old, independently wealthy, and the beneficiary of a generous, life-long pension from the government. However, he was entirely on his own, unmarried, unemployed, and uninterested in employment. What was he to do with his life?

To escape the scene of his humiliation as a lunatic, Minor moved to London and occupied himself with traveling, painting watercolors, and frequenting houses of prostitution. Most of the time, however, he struggled with his bad conscience. He felt tortured by what psychiatrists call "delusions" and "voices." One night, haunted by the terror of being pursued by one of his Irish tormentors, he shot to death a man he imagined was the malefactor. He made no effort to escape. When taken into custody, he apologized for his act: "It had been a terrible accident; he had shot the wrong man."[63]

From a legal point of view, the case was uncomplicated. Minor was a gentleman. He had been declared insane by the U.S. Army. He had been in an insane asylum in America. Obviously, he was not responsible for the murder. A judge impaneled a jury and instructed it to bring in a verdict of not guilty by reason of insanity. The jury obeyed, "without deliberation." On April 6, 1872, Minor was committed to "the newly built showpiece of the British penal system, a sprawling set of red-brick buildings located behind high walls and spiked fences in the village of Crowthorne, officially known as the Asylum for the Criminally Insane, Broadmoor."[64] In 1910, Minor was transferred to St. Elizabeths Hospital in Washington, D.C., and thence, in 1919, to the Retreat, an asylum in Hartford, Connecticut, near his nephew's home. He died in 1920, in his 85th year. His delusions—focused partly on seductive, naked Ceylonese women and partly on sinister, threatening Irish men—never left him.

This biographical sketch, excerpted from Simon Winchester's masterful account, *The Professor and the Madman*, is necessary background for understanding Minor's career as one of the builders of the *Oxford English Dictionary* (OED). At Broadmoor, "Minor was made more than just tolerably comfortable—not least because he was a well-born, well-educated man. And he had an income: All the Broadmoor officials knew he was a retired soldier, with a regular army pension paid by the United States government. So he was given not one cell but two, a pair of connecting rooms... There was an enchanting view..."[65]

Except for being deprived of a freedom for which Minor had no use, he could now live in comfort, with all his needs provided by paternalistic authorities and his own ample funds. He had his easel and paints, was allowed to hire fellow inmates to clean his rooms, and could purchase books and special foods. "William Minor was able to live a life of total leisure and security, he was warm and reasonably well fed, his health was attended to, he could stroll along the long gravel pathway known as the Terrace, he could take his ease on one of the benches by the lawn and gaze at the shrubbery, or he could read and paint to his heart's content." In short, his situation resembled that of a pampered child. Moreover—and here I must add something to Winchester's excellent account—Minor was not molested by an asylum staff eager to diagnose his illness or treat it. In those days, madness was widely accepted as a condition—indeed, a fate—termed a disease, but really not a disease at all.

As time passed, Minor approached the widow of the man he had murdered and apologized for his deed. She was a poor woman with two children. Minor began to use some of his money to support her. In turn, the woman became a kind of assistant to him, supplying him with books and other goods he wanted. Some time in the early 1880s, Minor came across a notice in a magazine, by Professor (later Sir) James Murray, asking for volunteers to help him in the construction of the OED. Murray wanted to create a very special dictionary. His aim was to enlist a large number of volunteers to read vast numbers of books and carefully record the meanings of words by means of illustrative phrases or sentences, tracing the development of each word from its oldest to its most up-to-date meanings.

Minor wrote to Murray offering his services. They began to collaborate. Minor quickly became one of the most valuable contributors to the project. Murray invited Minor to visit him at Oxford, an invitation Minor always declined, politely but without explanation. Mystified, Murray decided to visit his outstanding collaborator. When he arrived at Crowthorne and realized the address he was seeking was an insane asylum, he assumed he was about to meet its director. Murray and Minor met and became good friends. All the while, Minor's delusions continued to haunt him, especially at night. Yet, he did excellent work on the OED and was completely lucid. Winchester offers this account of the first meeting between Murray and Minor:

> It has been known for at least the last eighty years that among the scores of volunteers who helped contribute quotations to the OED, and who are listed in the great Preface to Volume 1, there was a murderer. He was named William Chester Minor, and he was a wealthy American surgeon-soldier who went mad when he was forced to brand a deserter during the Civil War. He came to England, uncured and incurable, and during a fit of madness shot a man dead. He was sentenced to be confined without parole in the newly-built Broadmoor Asylum for Criminal Lunatics in Crowthorne, Berkshire. It was while he was in his cell that Minor came across James Murray's famous Call for Volunteers, and decided, probably as a means of personal redemption, to begin work as a reader for the OED. Over the next thirty-eight years he contributed thousands upon thousands of quotations—prompting Murray once to say that "the supreme position is certainly held by Dr. W. C. Minor of Broadmoor. So enormous have been Dr. Minor's contributions...that we could easily illustrate the last four centuries from his quotations alone."[66]

Murray made several trips to Broadmoor. He recalled his visit in 1891 as follows: "I also wrote to Dr. Nicholson, then the Governor, who warmly invited me—and when I went, drove me from and to the Railway Station and invited me to lunch, at which he also had Dr. Minor, who I found was a great favorite with his children."[67] Murray also visited Minor in his rooms where, as if they had been in rooms at a college in Oxford, they shared tea: "It [the room] was lined with bookshelves, all of which were open except for one glass-fronted case that held the rarest of sixteenth- and seventeenth-century works from which much of the OED work was being done. The fireplace crackled merrily. Tea and Dundee cake were brought in by a fellow inmate whom Minor had hired to work for him."[68]

The scenes above illustrate how the meanings of terms such as "mental patient," "psychiatrist," and "mental hospital" have changed since 1890. I am confident that the present director of the Broadmoor hospital does not let an inmate hire another inmate to bring him tea, and that if he did such a thing, his colleagues would consider him mad and remove him from his position.

We hear much about "advances" in psychiatric diagnosis and treatment since the days when Minor was at Broadmoor. We hear nothing about what patients, psychiatrists, and society have lost in the process.

Robert Walser

Walser was born in the canton of Bern, the seventh of eight children. His father ran a store selling stationery and notions. At the age of fourteen, Robert was taken out of school and apprenticed to a bank. However, he had bigger ambitions. He wanted to become an actor. When his audition turned out to be a failure, he set his sights on becoming a writer. He moved to Berlin, wrote feverishly, and by the time he was thirty-one, he had several collections of poetry and three novels to his name, all of which were well received. His style, plain to the point of being considered "primitive," had a strong influence on the young Franz Kafka.

In 1913, Walser left Berlin and returned to Switzerland. He made a precarious living writing occasional pieces for newspapers, was depressed, and made an abortive suicide attempt. "It was suggested," writes South African novelist J. M. Coetzee, "that his sister should take him in, but she was unwilling. So he allowed himself to be committed to the sanatorium in Waldau... 'Responded evasively to questions about being sick of life,' ran the initial medical report. In later evaluations Walser's doctors would disagree about what, if anything, was wrong with him."[69]

There was nothing medically wrong with Walser. He just couldn't bear the struggle for existence that so-called normal life entails. Walser was a prophet for human insignificance, for being "small" to the point of social invisibility. The protagonist in his most famous novel, *Jakob von Gunten*, is a young man in an imaginary school devoted to giving its pupils an education in humility. The students aspire not to greatness, but smallness. Their goal is not self-expression, but self-effacement. "How fortunate I am," says the hero, "not to be able to see in myself anything worth respecting and watching! To be small and stay small."[70]

While residing in the asylum, Walser went for long walks and occupied himself with meaningless chores, like gluing paper bags. He told a visitor, "I'm not here to write. I'm here to be mad." To a friend he wrote: "One can do without much, and yet feel well... My illness is a disease of the head [Kopf], which is difficult to define. It is said to be incurable, but that does not hinder me from thinking about whatever I like, or to make calculations, or to write, or to have polite relations with people, or do things, e.g., have the satisfaction of a good meal, and so forth."[71]

Although diagnosed as schizophrenic, Walser remained lucid and in good general health. Long walks in the country remained his main activity. He was found dead on Christmas Day, 1956, frozen to death in a snowy field. He was seventy-eight years old. For the last forty-three years of his life, the insane asylum had been his home. In Zurich, a lane named *"Walser Gasse"* honors his memory.[72]

Respecting the Dignity of the Other

It is an old and wise observation that many people deemed mad are child-like—egotistical and conceited, yet at the same time over-sensitive to the suffering of others, shy and timid, and dependent on others. Like children, they are often incapable of asking for help directly, with words, partly because they feel it demeans them to do so, and partly to prevent being rebuffed. Instead, like children who cry rather than say they are tired and want to go to bed, mental patients ask for help with deeds, sometimes "mad," criminal deeds. Leonard I. Stein and Alberto B. Santos, two advocates of Assertive

Community Treatment, cite the example of a patient of theirs who made it a habit to secure admission to the mental hospital by brazenly stealing from supermarkets: "If he were not apprehended, he would simply walk back in and take more until someone called the police. He would then get into the police car and half a block down the road would say to the policeman, 'Oh, by the way, I'm a patient at the state hospital.' At this point, the policeman would sigh with relief..."[73]

Psychiatrists interpret unsuccessful suicide attempts as "cries for help." They ought to interpret unsuccessful criminal acts—that is, criminal acts that result in arrest—similarly, instead of dismissing them as the "senseless" acts of a mad person, "not responsible for his behavior." When a man with a long psychiatric record shoves a woman in front of a subway train, he probably does so, in part, because he wants room and board in a mental hospital. He knows that it is useless to ask for such a service, but that it is easily obtained by committing the appropriate crime. I am not saying that shoving a stranger in front of a subway train is a "simple" motivated act similar to going to a restaurant and ordering a meal to assuage one's hunger. The act may be a decision to yield to an impulse to cause harm or create a stir—an impulse such as we might all have on occasion. We easily resist such impulses. Individuals who yield to them do so for *reasons*.

By abolishing the asylum function of the madhouse, we have, albeit indirectly and unwittingly, encouraged, perhaps even compelled, certain desperate people to resort to desperate acts to secure the attention, food, and housing they need, but cannot or will not obtain for themselves.

I am not trying to romanticize the lost world of the insane asylum. It was no Eden. But there were valuable things in that world that we have lost, in particular, the respect that, by and large, patients had for psychiatrists, and vice versa. Most of the inmates of mental hospitals were bereft of family, social position, love, nearly everything—but the psychiatrist accepted the chronic mental patient for who he was. He was not expected to change, recover, become a "better" person. Today's chronic mental patient is just as bereft of family, social position, love, nearly everything, as van Gogh, Minor, and Walser had been—*and they are bereft of their right to be who they are as well.*

Vincent van Gogh and Robert Walser spent many years in mental hospitals, explicitly at their own request. William Chester Minor spent most of his life in mental hospitals, implicitly at his own request. While living in the asylum, van Gogh and Walser were free to come and go. Van Gogh socialized with the chief physician and painted his portrait. He regularly dined at a tavern, frequented houses of prostitution, and owned a gun. While in the fields painting, he shot himself to death. As a patient, Walser was not treated for his mental illness; instead, he was allowed to live as he wanted, keeping to himself, occupying himself mainly with long walks in the country. He was allowed to freeze to death.

Today, both mental patients and psychiatrists have much less freedom than they had fifty or a hundred years ago. Deprived of responsibility, dignity, and self-respect, patients are sentenced to boredom and uselessness. Held responsible for the destructive deeds of their patients, especially suicide and murder, psychiatrists are, in effect, prevented from having consensual relationships with them. At the same time, legal and professional expectations compel the psychiatrist to torment his patient with "treatments." In turn, the psychiatrist is subject to being terrorized by the patient, his family, and their lawyers. The patient is free to assault the psychiatrist physically and not be held responsible. The patient's family and lawyers are free to assault the psychiatrist with malpractice suits and the psychiatrist will be held liable for medical negligence.

When van Gogh killed himself, no one attributed his suicide to Dr. Gachet. Dr. Gachet did not force Vincent van Gogh to take drugs that would make his hands tremble and his body shake; nor did he do anything else to destroy van Gogh's ability to paint, feel, suffer, or kill himself. Dr. Gachet did not fear that he would be a target of Vincent's "aggression," or that he would lose his medical license for his failure to protect Vincent from killing himself, or that Theo would sue him for malpractice.

Walser died in 1956—not very long ago. Walser's life and death illustrate dramatically that, in Switzerland at least, some public mental hospitals still functioned as asylums, giving their patients a permanent home, without making them submit to unwanted treatments and without "deinstitutionalizing" them against their will. No state mental hospital director today would allow a committed patient to come and go as he pleased, as van Gogh and Walser had been allowed to do. No psychiatrist today could or would be willing to assume responsibility for the consequences of giving a patient such liberty as van Gogh and Walser enjoyed, or privileges such as Minor enjoyed.

An incident during Minor's stay at Broadmoor further illustrates how radically the psychiatric scene has changed during the past century. One day, Dr. Minor amputated his penis. Perhaps fearing that an imaginary surgeon might wish to reattach it, he threw his member into the fireplace. There is no need to belabor the contemporary legal and professional consequences, for the psychiatrist and the hospital, of a hospitalized mental patient cutting off his penis.

To be sure, the insane asylum was never intended to be *a true asylum* for patients. Alienists, jurists, and the public needed the institution for their own purposes, perhaps most importantly as evidence for the medical character of madness and the asylum doctor's *special expertise in diagnosing and managing it.*

Conclusions

An observer of the American social scene might conclude that Americans are obsessed with human rights and scientific medicine. Not so. They are obsessed with dependence on government for economic and medical security, to protect them from dangers they attribute to imaginary diseases.[74] This obsession is manifested by, among other things, Americans' increasing inability and unwillingness to distinguish between what is or ought to be the responsibility of others, especially doctors and the state, and what is or ought to remain the individual's own business.

"Should volunteering be mandatory?" runs the title of a piece in the *Los Angeles Times* on March 31, 2001.[75] According to Betsy Alkaly, community service program administrator for the Venice (California) High School, high school students ought to be required to perform volunteer services to qualify for graduation: "Is it contradictory to make volunteer work mandatory?" she asks. No: "Sometimes as educators we have to require students to do things they should do voluntarily. And in this instance, *it's something that is good for the students, good for the community, and good for the school.*"[76] This is not true; if it were, there would be no need for coercion.

The rhetoric of coercive psychiatric therapy reprises the rhetoric of forcible religious conversion and the rhetoric of chattel slavery. The formula is: "We, the authorities, are your benefactors. We know that you need X and that X is good for you. Hence, if we force you to believe, do, or ingest X, we are only facilitating your voluntary behavior and advancing your own best interests."

The result is that liberals and conservatives, Democrats and Republicans, jurists and journalists—all agree that the only good mental patient is the mental patient "on medication." The picture looks very different to anyone who believes that *forcing people to take drugs to change their behavior is not treatment.* However, since most mental health professionals and most of the public believe the opposite, implementing outpatient commitment and investigating its effectiveness are big business.

8

Glorifying Psychiatric Slavery:
Therapeutic Jurisprudence

Take up the White Man's burden, send forth the best ye breed,...
To serve your captives' need; to wait, in heavy harness
On fluttered folk and wild, your new-caught sullen peoples,
Half devil and half child...
Take up the White Man's burden, and reap his old reward,
The blame of those ye better, the hate of those ye guard...
—Rudyard Kipling (1865-1936)[1]

Slave camps under the flag of freedom, massacres justified by philanthropy, or by the taste for the superhuman, in one sense cripple judgment. On the day when crime dons the apparel of innocence—through a curious transposition peculiar to our times—it is innocence that is called upon to justify itself.
—Albert Camus (1913-1960)[2]

The history of the modern West is littered with the carcasses of violent and unjust acts on which we now look back in horror. Chattel slavery, the disfranchisement of women, Christian anti-Semitism and the Holocaust, the incarceration of Japanese-Americans after Pearl Harbor, and the persecution of homosexuals is just a sample of the major acts of collective violence and injustice that the modern Western mind—moralizing with a backward gaze—now condemns as crimes against humanity.

Alexis de Tocqueville rightly observed: "To commit violent and unjust acts, it is not enough for a government to have the will or even the power; the habits, ideas, and passions of the time must lend themselves to their committal."[3] Tocqueville might have added that collective violence and injustice are also justified by the law. That assertion, albeit seemingly paradoxical, is actually a tautology. What does the law represent if not the "habits, ideas, and passions of the

147

time"? *It is the task of the legal profession to justify justice, and hence also injustice.*[4] The mutating legal justifications for psychiatric coercion form an integral part of the history of psychiatric slavery.

"Who would believe," laments Nobel Laureate Milton Friedman, "that a democratic government would pursue for eight decades a failed policy that produced tens of millions of victims and trillions of dollars of illicit profits for drug dealers; cost taxpayers hundreds of billions of dollars; increased crime and destroyed inner cities; fostered wide-spread corruption and violations of human rights—and all with no success in achieving the stated and unattainable objective of a drug-free America?"[5] It is a rhetorical question. The public perceives the violence and injustice of the war on drugs—and on mental illness—as neither violent nor unjust, but the very opposite: therapeutic and just.

In this chapter I show how the rebirth of an undivided psychiatry, facilitated by a reductionist neuroscience and a corrupt psychopharmacology, was promoted and justified by a new philosophy of jurisprudence, aptly named "therapeutic."

A Brief History of Neuropsychiatry

Early mad-doctoring rested on a primitive sort of neuropsychiatry. Insanity was assumed to be, and was defined as, a product of brain disease. From the end of the seventeenth until the end of nineteenth century, neuropsychiatry, based on that unquestioned premise, was a house undivided. If a person was considered truly crazy, he was regarded as unfit for liberty and was confined in an insane asylum. Prior to 1900, the professional practices we know as "outpatient psychiatry" or "office psychotherapy" did not exist. While some persons not confined in mental hospitals were viewed as eccentric or odd, they were considered neither mad nor ill, and no one proposed limiting their liberty by mental health laws.

Psychiatry and Neurology: Divorce and Remarriage

The works of Pierre Janet in France, Sigmund Freud in Austria, and Carl Jung in Switzerland split psychiatry in two. Patients suffering from serious mental diseases, who were called "psychotics," were incarcerated in mental hospitals and continued to occupy the status of psychiatric slaves. Patients suffering from less serious forms of mental diseases, who were called "neurotics," were "treated" as voluntary patients by psychiatrists and nonmedical psychotherapists and occupied the same status as medical patients or non-patients. An old joke satirized psychiatry as follows: "The neurotic builds castles in the air. The psychotic lives in them. And the psychiatrist collects the rent."

The point to keep in mind is that so-called neurotics resided in their own homes, paid for the psychiatric services they received, and retained their civil rights and duties. Sometimes, the neurotic patient, especially if he was wealthy and suffered from "alcoholism" or "neurasthenia," checked himself into a "sanatorium," where he was treated as both guest and patient, catered to round the clock by medical and nonmedical personnel at his beck and call. When the patient decided he had enough treatment, he paid the bill and left. In *Tender is the Night,* F. Scott Fitzgerald gave a memorable description of the inner workings of such sanatoria.

From the end of World War I to the introduction of psychotropic drugs in the 1950s, psychiatry was a house divided, inhabited by two different kinds of psychiatrists. One group consisted of psychiatrists who were state employees: their job was to "care" for the patients sent to the hospitals by relatives and judges. The patients resided in state mental hospitals, were confined against their will, did not initiate and could not terminate their relationship with psychiatrists. Another group consisted of psychiatrists who practiced on the model of regular physicians: their job was to help patients who sought their services. The patients lived in their own homes or wherever they pleased, initiated and terminated their relationship with psychiatrists, and paid for the services they received.

That was the case, at least in principle. In practice, the separation was never quite so clean. A substantial number of psychoanalysts limited their practices to voluntary office patients, while others engaged in coercive hospital practices as well. Similarly, many state hospital psychiatrists maintained private office practices with voluntary outpatients.

For about forty years, from 1920 to 1960, the private practice of psychotherapy/psychoanalysis flourished in the United States.[6] During the next forty years, it steadily declined. The reversal was due partly to the events outlined above, and partly to radical changes in the economics of medical practice. In 1950, patients receiving psychotherapy paid for the service out of their own pockets. Fifty years later, health insurance companies pay for it, even when the service is rendered by psychologists or social workers. (Fifty years ago, members of those professions were legally prohibited from rendering mental health services as independent contractors.)

Still, human relations that resemble what used to be considered voluntary private psychiatric treatments flourish. Millions of Americans seek and receive the services of "therapists," a class that now includes not only psychiatrists, psychologists, and social workers, but also addiction specialists, philosophers, and counselors of every imaginable kind. However, severing the direct economic connection between therapist and patient inevitably entails that both parties lose the power to define the parameters of the service requested and rendered. No longer can these two parties contract freely for "therapy." For example, the patient who speaks of suicide runs the risk of being involuntarily hospitalized; similarly, the psychiatrist who refrains from prescribing drugs runs the risk of being sued for malpractice.

The novel rights of patients and the novel duties of psychiatrists led to the creation of what judges called the "special therapeutic relationship": the psychotherapeutic situation was transformed, from a *private contractual relationship* between two responsible adults into a *public status relationship* between a guardian and his ward.

In the 1950s, the therapist was an agent of his patient. Today, he is a double agent, with triple duties: a duty to the patient for "treatment," broadly defined; a duty to the state, imposed by law and psychiatric ethics, to protect the patient from himself and the public from the patient; and a duty to third parties—such as spouses, children, and friends of the patient—to notify them as soon as he has reason to believe that a patient is dangerous specifically to them.

The result is that the patient cannot trust the therapist, and the therapist cannot keep the patient's communications confidential. What had been an alliance between a patient-buyer and a therapist-seller engaged in a common enterprise, has been transformed into a conflict of interests, creating an antagonism between a citizen-client entitled to a service and a therapist-agent of the state obligated to conduct himself in conformity with his job description.

In the 1950s, when I started to publish a series of articles in professional journals on the relationship between law and psychiatry, I had hoped that my efforts might lead to a separation of voluntary psychiatry from involuntary psychiatry.[7] The opposite has happened. Critiquing the concept of mental illness and questioning the moral legitimacy of psychiatric coercions and excuses led to a powerful professional reaction, the *"remedicalization" of psychiatry*, and a vigorous judicial-legislative activism, *validating psychiatry's identity as a medical specialty and the moral legitimacy of psychiatric coercions as treatments.*[8] Aided and abetted by the government and the media, the dogmatic declaration that certain behaviors are medical maladies was accepted as proof that they are *bona fide* diseases, resulting from chemical imbalances in the brain. This claim, in turn, justified the use of a new class of drugs designed to cure mental illnesses. With circular logic, the very use of "psychiatric drugs" supported the belief that mental diseases are brain diseases. At long last, psychiatrists appeared to resemble other physicians: they observed behaviors and claimed that they were based on brain diseases; then they attached diagnostic labels to them, declared them to be diseases, and prescribed drugs as treatments for them.

At least for now, the psychopharmacologists have managed to heal the breach in psychiatry created by the pioneer psychotherapists a century earlier. Rationalized as brain science and validated as pharmacological treatment, psychiatric slavery rules undisputed. However, the belief that mental diseases are curable with antidepressants and antipsychotics is founded on faith, not fact. Hence, policies based on it are destined to fail. In 1956, when news of tranquilizing drugs first appeared in the psychiatric literature, I cautioned that they "function as chemical straitjackets... When patients had to be restrained by the use of [physical] force—for example, by a straitjacket—it was difficult for those in charge of their care to convince themselves that they were acting altogether on behalf of the patient... Restraint by chemical means does not make [others] feel guilty; herein lies the danger to the patient."[9]

Far from making psychiatrists feel guilty, restraining patients by chemical means emboldened them to make the use of psychiatric drugs in effect compulsory for both mental patients and psychiatrists. "Talk therapy" is now relegated to psychologists and social workers. Psychiatrists are expected to make diagnoses and prescribe and monitor medications. This expectation meshes with, and is reinforced by, most people's deep-seated craving for "medications": some people love to take psychiatric drugs for their pharmacological effects; others, because it validates their status as sick patients. Also, when mental patients take prescribed psychoactive drugs it reassures relatives, employers, friends, and the public that dangerous persons are being rendered harmless. Being "on medication" becomes synonymous with being in control of oneself, or being properly controlled by competent experts, making patients and nonpatients alike feel that all is well in the world.

Law and the Mental Patient: Who Benefits?

Life in modern Western societies, nowhere more than in the United States, is regulated by law. This has made the legal profession especially important, as both friend and foe of liberty. No lawyer declares that he is against civil rights. The term "civil rights," like the term "health," has become simply an honorific appellation, lacking any specific content. The important thing for a speaker or writer is making sure that he does not to appear to be against it. How, then, do lawyers oppose civil rights? By defining their support of what I regard as civil wrongs—specifically, psychiatric slavery—as serving the best interests of the disfranchised persons. As this legal tactic caters to the interests of the legal and medical professions as well as to the public, the destroyers of liberty are celebrated as its defenders.

More than forty years have passed since Erving Goffman and I lamented the spectacle of the so-called civil libertarian supporting psychiatric slavery. In a series of law review articles published in the 1950s and 1960s, I criticized the legal profession for its uncritical acceptance of psychiatric deprivations of individual liberty and personal responsibility.[10] In 1961, Goffman observed: "It is an odd historical fact that persons concerned with promoting civil liberties in other areas of life tend to favor giving the psychiatrist complete discretionary power over the patient. Apparently it is felt that the more power possessed by medically qualified administrators and therapists, the better the interests of the patients will be served."[11]

In 1971, George Alexander, professor of law at Santa Clara University, Erving Goffman, and I founded the American Association for the Abolition of Involuntary Mental Hospitalization (AAAIMH).[12] Our aim was to give voice to psychiatric abolitionists from all walks of life and assist psychiatric slaves to regain their freedom. Nine years later, realizing that our small group, lacking access to funds and the media, was not up to this task, we abandoned the effort.[13] Professional and popular opinion were running in the opposite direction. The forces of therapeutic jurisprudence had won the hearts and minds of America's leading opinion-makers and of the American people.

Krafft-Ebing, Freud, and Legal Psychiatry

The policy of using the coercive apparatus of the state as if it were a type of medical therapy is as old as psychiatry itself. Toward the end of the nineteenth century, the view that it is the proper function of psychiatry to set and enforce public policy regarding personal behaviors formerly considered sinful became a veritable ideology. The two major figures whose work laid the foundations for the cultural-legal transformation of sexual sins and crimes into mental illnesses were Baron Richard von Krafft-Ebing (1840-1902), professor of psychiatry at the University of Vienna, and Sigmund Freud (1856-1939).

Krafft-Ebing owes much of his fame to a single book, *Psychopathia Sexualis*. First published in 1886, this work went through numerous editions in German and became an international best seller. In retrospect, it is obvious why this book became so vastly popular. It was the first modern pornographic tract successfully merchandised as a medical text, a feat accomplished by larding it with Latin words. Given that in those days most educated people had a working knowledge of Latin, this must have made the book all the more titillating.

Prior to the publication of *Psychopathia Sexualis*, abnormal sexual acts were, literally, "unspeakable abominations," shoved under the carpet of human consciousness as bestial, unnatural, and, of course, at once sinful and criminal. Thus, the law and society could not turn their backs on what were then, in a telling conflation of sin and sickness, called "perversions." Krafft-Ebing's text was, in effect, a menu of forbidden sexual pleasures and a manual on how to perform them. In our day, many of these acts have been "discovered" to be basic human rights and, of course, essential tools of "sex therapy."[14] The alleged diseases Krafft-Ebing identified as "Cerebral Neuroses" included: *"Anaesthesia* (absence of sexual instinct)... *Hyperaesthesia* (increased desire, satyriasis)... *Paraesthesia* (perversion of the sexual instinct)... *Sadism* (the association of lust and cruelty)... *Masochism* is the counterpart of sadism... *Fetishism* invests imaginary presentations of separate parts of the body or portions of raiment of the opposite sex...with voluptuous sensations."[15]

Why did Krafft-Ebing write *Psychopathia Sexualis*? "The object of this treatise," he claimed, "is merely to record the various psycho-pathological manifestations of sexual life in man... The physician finds, perhaps, a solace in the fact that he may at times refer those manifestations which offend against our ethical and aesthetical principles to a diseased condition of the mind or the body."[16] Krafft-Ebing did not merely want to record a variety of sexual acts. He wanted to medicalize and psychopathologize them, in order to remove them from the realm of jurisprudence and criminal law and transfer them to the realm of psychiatry and mental health law: "The medical barrister only then finds out how sad the lack of our knowledge is in the domain of sexuality when he is called upon to express an opinion as to the responsibility of the accused whose life, liberty, and honor are at stake."[17] Note that Krafft-Ebing identified his role as that of a "medical barrister." He did not claim that he was making a neuropathological diagnosis or was treating a patient.

If an act is defined as a crime and is prohibited by criminal law, and if a person commits that act, is caught, and is brought to trial, what role should the physician play in the adjudication of that person's guilt or innocence? The answer hinges on whether the act is perceived and defined as *caused,* partly or wholly, by a disease from which the defendant suffers. If the act is viewed as having nothing to do with disease—today few such acts remain—then doctors have no rational role in the trial. On the other hand, if the act is viewed as being a direct manifestation or "product" of a disease—the "meaningless" violence of a "diagnosed schizophrenic"—then doctors have a decisive role to play in it.

One of the main architects of the modern—outwardly scientific, but actually pseudoscientific—perception of misbehavior as mental illness was Krafft-Ebing. He declared: "The physician finds, perhaps, a solace in the fact that he may at times refer those manifestations which offend against our ethical or aesthetical principles to a diseased condition of the mind or the body. He can save the honor of humanity in the forum of morality, and the honor of the individual before the judge and his fellow-men. It is from the search of truth that the exalted duties and *rights of medical science* emanate."[18] Again, the speaker's language reveals his intent: Krafft-Ebing speaks of the "rights of medical science," by which he means the rights of psychiatry. Political philosophy and the law are supposed to be concerned with the *rights of the individual*, not the *rights of medical science*.

Freud's work is familiar and I will not say much about it here. I shall limit myself to calling attention to his message, both explicit and implicit, in *The Psychopathology of Everyday Life* (1901).[19] Recognizing that the behaviors of persons considered mentally abnormal are "governed" by the same principles that "govern" the behavior of persons considered mentally normal, Freud had two choices. He could have concluded, with Shakespeare, that "there is method in madness" and that there is no mental illness. He could then have written about the "normality of mentally ill persons" and their rights. Instead, Freud concluded that mentally healthy persons resemble mentally ill persons and wrote about the abnormality of mentally healthy persons: the phrase "the psychopathology of everyday life" successfully insinuated that normal behavior is similar to abnormal behavior, that every one is (more or less) mentally ill, and ought to be viewed as such.[20] As we know, this perspective became the basis for modern psychiatry.[21]

How did Freud demonstrate that mentally healthy behaviors resemble mentally sick behaviors? By claiming "complete psychical determinism" for both: "If the distinction between conscious and unconscious motivation is taken into account, our feeling of conviction informs us that conscious motivation does not extend to all our motor decisions...what is thus left free by the one side receives its motivation from the other side, from the unconscious; and in this way determination in the psychical sphere is still carried out without any gap."[22] Note Freud's use of pompous but vacuous phrases such as "psychical determinism," "our conviction informs us," and "motor decisions." Where, as we might now say, was Freud going with such ideas? Toward destroying the rule of law and hence liberty. In a revealing footnote added in 1907, he proudly stated: "These conceptions of the strict determination of apparently arbitrary psychical acts have already borne rich fruit... [Freud then cites the work of two criminologists who] have developed...a *technique* for the establishment of the facts of criminal proceedings."[23] These techniques were and are nothing but the biased and bought opinions of psychiatrists as agents of a party to a conflict, usually the state.[24]

Neither Krafft-Ebing nor Freud invented the idea that ordinary behaviors, condemned by some religions as sins, are, "in fact," mental diseases. No particular person invented it. The idea is an integral part of the phenomenon we call the Enlightenment, characterized by a shift from a religious to a scientific-pseudoscientific outlook on life. Since science is not doctrinal, there is, and can be, no absolute authority to answer questions such as, "Who speaks for science?" or "Who is authorized to distinguish science from pseudoscience?" Science and pseudoscience flourish together; and, because an attack on one is an attack on the other, perish together.

The most influential system of modern pseudoscience is psychiatry and psychoanalysis.[25] For present purposes, it is enough to understand how the psychiatric-pseudoscientific interpretation of ordinary sexual acts, epitomized by masturbation, laid the ground for making psychiatry a part of the modern state's legal system of behavior control.

Throughout the twentieth century, psychiatrists and psychoanalysts pursued Krafft-Ebing's agenda, creating what I have called a therapeutic state, regulating unwanted behaviors by pharmacratic, rather than legal, controls.[26] This is the background against which so-called therapeutic jurisprudence ought to be viewed.

Therapeutic Jurisprudence

The term "therapeutic jurisprudence" is the creation of David B. Wexler and Bruce J. Winick, professors of law at the University of Arizona, in Tucson, and the University of Miami, respectively. They define it as "the study of the role of the law as a therapeutic agent."[27] At best, this claim is a half-truth. In fact, therapeutic jurisprudence is not about studying the law, it is about perverting the law by promoting psychiatric slavery. Wexler and Winick themselves acknowledge that they seek to apply "the knowledge, theories, and insights of the mental health and related disciplines [to] shape the development of the law."[28]

I submit that therapeutic jurisprudence stands in the same relation to justice as antebellum judicial opinion about slavery stood to justice. In his seminal book, A Peculiar Humanism, William E. Wiethoff, professor of speech and communication at Indiana University, relates how Southern judges "told again and again an archetypal fable in which enlightened masters improved the lot of Africans by removing them from a savage existence, satisfying their basic needs, and introducing them to Christianity."[29]

The advocates of therapeutic jurisprudence tell a similar, though less ancient, fable, in which enlightened psychiatrists improve the lot of mental patients by removing them from the responsibilities of life, satisfying their basic needs, and providing them with "therapy." In short, therapeutic jurisprudence is the name of a system of *legal apologetics for justifying psychiatric slavery in particular, and the therapeutic state in general.*

The legal justification of slavery rested on the denial that slave law dealt with master and slave in conflict with one another, and that what one party experienced as help, the other was likely to experience as harm. In 1856, Josiah J. Evans, a South Carolina judge, told the United States Senate: "In relation to the African, no man in this House, and no man out of it, can say that there is any corner of this earth, upon which the African race are as well off, as well provided for, with more of the elements of happiness that in the slave parts of the United States."[30] Therapeutic jurisprudence rests on a similar denial, that is, the denial that mental health law deals with psychiatrist and involuntary mental patient in conflict with one another, and that what one party calls "help," the other experiences as harm.

Proslavery writers insisted on denying that the relationship between master and slave was intrinsically adversarial and represented it as paternal. Pro-psychiatric slavery writers insist on denying that the relationship between psychiatrist and involuntary psychiatric patient is intrinsically adversarial and represent it as therapeutic. This denial underlies everything Wexler and Winick say. For example, they state that "therapeutic jurisprudence is the use of social science to study the extent to which a legal rule or practice promotes the psychological or physical well-being of the people it affects."[31] Which people? The psychiatric slaveholder or the psychiatric slave?

Ignoring the French maxim, *Qui s'excuse, s'accuse* (He who excuses himself, accuses himself), Winick anticipates the accusation that he supports psychiatric coercions and tries to refute it. "My work," he states, "has praised the law's commitment to the principle of individual autonomy on the basis that self-determination is therapeutically advantageous... Legal protection for individual autonomy can have positive therapeutic value."[32] This is both wrong and wrongheaded. Self-determination is not therapeutically advantageous for everyone, under all circumstances: the prisoner or committed mental patient is likely to fare better if he obeys orders than if he exercises self-determination. Secondly, autonomy and self-determination are values because they are essential aspects of individual liberty, regardless of whether they have a "positive therapeutic advantage": the prisoner on a hunger strike may die, which is hardly a therapeutic advantage, but he is exercising autonomy and self-determination.

In addition to promoting psychiatric slavery, Winick supports all the fashionable agendas of left-liberal statists. Regarding gun controls, he writes: "Were comparative therapeutic jurisprudence research in a society that bans handguns to demonstrate significant positive consequences to mental and physical health, this research might prompt clarification of the Second Amendment's reach and pave the way for legislative action."[33] The translation of this jargon into English would read: let us do a study to prove that gun controls are therapeutic and use it to support legislation to ban guns. The researcher into therapeutic jurisprudence is not supposed to entertain the possibility that people might regard having a right to own a gun as therapeutic and that no contrived study can resolve the controversy regarding this issue.

Ironically, much of my work during the past forty years may be read as a systematic critique of therapeutic jurisprudence.[34] It is possible that my writings concerning legal psychiatry, like early abolitionist literature, stimulated a more vigorous defense of the institution under attack. Classical liberals consider imprecision with respect to what counts as crime and punishment incompatible with the rule of law; whereas modern liberals consider imprecision with respect to what counts as mental illness and psychiatric treatment as its most distinctive and valuable feature. "In defining 'therapeutic' broadly to include anything that enhances the psychological or physical well-being of the individual," writes Winick, "therapeutic jurisprudence has left the concept of 'therapeutic' ambiguous and open to argument about what should count as therapeutic... At the core of the concept is the concern for avoiding or ameliorating *psychopathology in the traditional sense.*"[35]

We call a thing a "key" only if it can open a "lock." As key implies lock, so therapy implies illness. Winick's view illustrates a commitment to the broadly flexible, metaphoric use of the words "illness" and "therapy," characteristic of their uses in psychiatry. Although Winick disclaims promoting psychiatric slavery, that is precisely what he does: "If recognition of the right [to refuse psychiatric treatment]...could be shown to cause serious harm to those with mental illness who might assert it, then concern for beneficence might lead courts and legislators to deny the right in certain circumstances or to construe it narrowly."[36] Apologists for slavery also claimed to be motivated by beneficence. "For hard-pressed judges," writes Wiethoff, "the humanist defense of slavery was attractive because it was well defined and grounded in traditional principles... Tragically, the judges did not tell the truth about slavery... Instead they narrated their intuitions and their idealized lifestyles."[37]

Winick does not consider the possibility of the patient's having a guardian who could refuse treatment on his behalf. In the Introduction, I cited Stephen Rachlin's view that the mental patient should never have the right to refuse treatment: "the right to refuse treatment is one right too many."[38] That is the posture of the psychiatric slaveholder: the slave can never have a right to self-determination.

In contrast, I maintain that—regardless of the nature of the "condition" a psychiatric diagnosis ostensibly identifies—every adult, unless declared legally incompetent, should have an unqualified right to reject psychiatric treatment. If he has been declared incompetent (or is a minor), then his guardian should have an unqualified right to reject psychiatric treatment on his behalf. The psychiatrist may, of course, retain the privilege to recommend the treatment he believes the patient needs; but, in a free society, under no circumstances should the psychiatrist have the right to impose treatment on the patient, against his express wishes or the express wishes of his guardian. As matters stand, for all practical purposes the psychiatrist has such a right, which places him squarely in the role of a slave owner with a right to dispose at will over the "welfare" of his slave.

The glorification of chattel slavery on the eve of the Civil War was no doubt useful for blinding the slaveholders to the brutalities of slavery. But it inflamed the abolitionists. The glorification of psychiatric slavery today has had a similar effect on me. I end this chapter with a brief review of the theory and practice of psychiatric brutalities, as described by their proud practitioners.

The Theory and Practice of Psychiatric Violence

Before World War II, many state mental hospitals were known as "snake pits," warehousing thousands of mental patients in filthy "back wards." Yet, psychiatrists were not afraid of the patients, largely, I believe, because they left the patients alone. Today, mental hospitals are "treatment units," housing a small number of patients in reasonably clean quarters. And psychiatrists are afraid of the patients, mainly, I believe, because they harass them with so-called treatments that make the patients feel existentially castrated. One of the most violent places in America today is the ward of a mental hospital. According to Kenneth Tardiff, professor of psychiatry at Cornell, in two "highly staffed treatment units," one aggressive act occurred every half-hour of working time.[39]

Psychiatric Violence as Medical Treatment

The premise behind the creation of the profession of mad-doctoring was that the insane person is "mad," "furious," a "savage beast." He must be restrained for his own welfare and for the safety of the community. The control of violence, however, is supposed to be a function of the police. Why, then, do policemen not perform this function? There are two closely connected answers to this question. One is because the violence appears to be bizarre or irrational, for example, the killing of a stranger. Psychiatrists usually call the person who engages in such conduct an "insane criminal" or "criminally insane." The other is because the violence is directed against the individual himself, for example, self-starvation or suicide. Psychiatrists typically call the person who engages in such conduct "psychotic" or "mentally ill and dangerous to himself." Neither of these two types of actions or persons fits the traditional concept of the criminal as a person engaging in what appears to be a rationally motivated, goal-directed type of behavior, exemplified by the man who robs a bank.

When we call violence against others "senseless," we deny the self-evident, albeit unusual, rationality of the act. When we call violence against the self "senseless," *we refuse to be satisfied with offering to help the person.* Although the person who commits violence against others commits a crime, whereas the person who violates himself does not, we blur and indeed obliterate this difference and treat members of both groups as if they belong in the same class: the severely mentally ill.

By viewing such diverse behaviors through psychiatry-colored lenses, we prevent ourselves from responding to the problems they present in any way other than by psychiatric repression and violence. The insane criminal appears to us as too different from the sane criminal—mad rather than just bad. The suicidal patient appears to us as too different from the ordinary patient—bad rather than just mad. Moreover, since we perceive his behavior as a kind of self-punishment, how can we punish him?[40] The result is that we refuse to punish the criminals and refuse to abstain from punishing the innocent. We therefore destroy the differences between these two kinds of behaviors and persons, whose only common feature is that they upset us, and control both as "dangerous mental patients," by means of psychiatric sanctions. This blurring of the boundary between crime and vexation, and the control of both the lawbreaker and the vexatious person by means of psychiatric controls, is the basic mandate of modern psychiatry.

The Rhetoric of Psychiatric Violence

I showed earlier that the language in which the practice of psychiatric coercion is couched legitimizes the violence. When chemical straitjackets are not enough to pacify patients, psychiatrists turn to seclusion and physical restraints as "therapeutic modalities."

The editors of *The Psychiatric Uses of Seclusion and Restraint,* Thomas G. Gutheil and Kenneth Tardiff, write: "Seclusion of the patient may be indicated for both the patient's benefit and that of the environment."[41] They and other psychiatrists pontificate about the "indications and contraindications for seclusion and restraint" as if these measures were real medical treatments, ignoring that most patients so managed are *legally competent*, making psychiatric aggression against them, by definition, assault, not treatment. Instead of arrest by the police and prosecution by the district attorney, competent patients who assault others are defined by psychiatrists as having a "psychiatric emergency," which justifies psychiatric counterviolence as "emergency treatment."

In a memorable poem, Kipling satirized the colonist's beneficent violence against the natives as "the white man's burden." Chattel slavery was another case of the white man's burden. Psychiatric slavery is the "psychiatrist's burden," a modern "therapeutic" version of beneficent oppression, leading to liberation in an ever-receding future.

The advocates of therapeutic jurisprudence unreservedly support the psychiatrist's systematic violence against the mental patient. Wexler states approvingly that psychiatrists "possess a great deal of leeway in administering seclusion and restraints in emergency situations."[42] Appealing to an emergency to justify the arbitrary use of force has always been the favorite tactic of the tyrant. Any emergency will do: it does not matter whether it is an economic, epidemiological, national, or psychiatric emergency.

Yet, some of the writers of pro-slavery apologetics knew that there was something fundamentally phony about their stand, and so do some of the writers of pro-psychiatric slavery. Joshua G. Clarke, a judge in antebellum Mississippi, feeling compelled to defend slavery, pleaded that "villains, in England, were more degraded than our slaves...[but] wanted his potential critics to appreciate his distress." [43] Tardiff is also defensive, feebly claiming that it is the psychiatrists, not just the patients, who are oppressed. He writes: "The need to control and contain disturbed and violent behavior remains the principal reason for the persistence of seclusion and restraint in the modern milieu as in the past... We have no cures for violence, yet social forces outside the profession direct our effort toward the care of violent patients in ever-growing numbers. Social policy decisions, legislative funding priorities, and rising social expectations have increased the visibility of violent patients and the demands that the mental health profession deal with them."[44]

This is an excuse, not an explanation. Psychiatrists are not soldiers. They cannot credibly claim that they are "only following orders." Psychiatrists are free moral agents. If they truly don't like the orders society gives their profession, they could make a concerted effort to change the orders. They could try to persuade society to let psychiatrists, like other physicians, be responsible for treating only voluntary patients. But they have never tried to do so. They have never rejected coercion in principle, or in practice. Today, with ever-increasing vehemence, they embrace it as a form of genuine medical treatment. Yet, Tardiff complains that psychiatrists are *compelled* to treat more and more Americans as psychiatric slaves: "Rising social expectations concerning the ability of mental health professionals to deal with disruptive behavior have encouraged the redefinition of alcohol-related offenses and of family violence as symptoms of emotional illness rather than criminal offenses."[45]

Most persons, especially persons innocent of lawbreaking, experience their forcible incarceration under psychiatric auspices as naked aggression against them. They believe that it is the psychiatrists who are "dangerous" and "violent," and psychiatrists know this. That is why they insist that "seclusion is a highly respected form of treatment, of great value to many severely disturbed patients."[46] The psychiatrist's belief that depriving an innocent person of liberty is "life-saving treatment" explains not only why he stubbornly defends psychiatric violence, but also why he perceives those who oppose his "benevolence" as profoundly immoral.

Conclusions

The forcible drug treatment of mental patients is a hallmark of psychiatric aggression, violence masquerading as therapy. Deinstitutionalization, the *de facto* forcible expulsion of the mental patient from the hospital that has become his home, compounds the problem. These acts of psychiatric violence generate counter-violence among the patients. At the same time, the only ticket that guarantees a patient admission to a mental hospital is violence, that is, the display of dangerousness to self or others. In effect, modern practices of psychiatric slavery are a system based on violence, by both patients and psychiatrists.

It is a truism that individuals as well as governments justify their aggression as self-defense. No one acknowledges that he initiates violence. Everyone believes that he only responds to it.[47] Reflecting on wars to do good, C. S. Lewis concluded that the do-gooder is the guilty aggressor. He famously warned: "Of all the tyrannies a tyranny sincerely exercised for the good of the victims may be the most oppressive... To be 'cured' against one's will and cured of states which we may not even regard as disease is to be put on a level with those who have not yet reached the age of reason or those who never will; to be classed with infants, imbeciles, and domestic animals."[48]

Lewis feared that a therapeutic tyrant would reduce people to the status of domestic animals. The modern humanitarian, imbued with the zeal of therapeutic jurisprudence, goes even further: he reduces persons he calls "mentally ill" to the status of stones. Michael S. Moore, professor of law and professor of philosophy at the University of San Diego, writes: "It is not so much that we excuse them [the mentally ill] from a *prima facie* case of responsibility; rather, by being unable to regard them as fully rational beings, we cannot affirm the essential condition to viewing them as moral agents to begin with. In this the mentally ill join (to a decreasing degree) infants, wild beasts, plants, and stones—none of which are responsible because of the absence of any assumption of rationality."[49]

History will be the judge.

Epilogue: "Liberty is the Prevention of Control by Others"[1]

I cannot accept your canon that we are to judge Pope and King unlike other men, with a favorable presumption that they did no wrong. If there is any presumption it is the other way against the holders of power, increasing as the power increases. Historic responsibility has to make up for want of legal responsibility. Power tends to corrupt and absolute power corrupts absolutely... There is no worse heresy than that the office sanctifies the holder of it.

—*Lord Acton (1834-1902)*[2]

Fallacies do not cease to be fallacies because they become fashions.
—*Gilbert K. Chesterton (1874-1936)*[3]

The longer I live, the more deeply impressed I am by the repetitive character of certain patterns of behavior, both individual and collective. Perhaps nowhere is this more apparent than in the forcible subjection of man by man in the name of benevolence and liberation, in short, coercive paternalism. Masters, aristocrats, priests, politicians, physicians at the top; slaves, serfs, women, sick persons, mental patients at the bottom.

Historically, the relationship between "liberator" and "liberated" resembles the children's game of musical chairs, which aptly symbolizes a fundamental principle of social organization. Regardless of the identity of the players, the result is always the same: winning means excluding the Other.

The real-life game of excluding requires authority or power or, preferably, both. The most effective excluders, therefore, have been church and state, separately and especially in combination. "Both Rome and Judea taught the union of church and state," warned Lord Acton.[4] Uniquely, the United States was founded on the principle that church and state ought to be disunited and stay forever separate. Nominally, this has been successfully accomplished. Unfortunately, the situation is not quite so simple. In the course of the past

half century, our democratic republic has, in effect, become transformed into a pharmacratic autocracy, based on the union of medicine and the state.[5] In its intolerance of deviants, modern American
pharmacracy rivals the medieval theocracies. To be sure, the ex-
cluded Other is not the religious heretic, but the medical heretic.

"Democracy," Acton continued, "has been known to cherish slavery, imperialism, wars of conquest, religious intolerance, tyranny,
equality in ignorance... Democracy has no means of putting down
opinion. If the opinion of society is corrupt, it cannot punish acts
which a body of opinion approves. Its juries would sympathize with
the malefactor."[6] When the body of opinion approved of religious
wars, its juries sympathized with the religious warriors, not their victims. Today, when the body of opinion approves of wars on drugs
and mental diseases, its juries sympathize with the medical warriors,
not their victims. Acton would have expected and predicted that,
regardless of how many "rights" we "give" mental patients, as long
as coercive psychiatric principles and practices receive political, professional, and popular support, the lot of individuals labeled as mentally ill will remain the same or worsen.

All my professional life I have opposed the basic principles and
practices of psychiatry—mental illness, civil commitment, and the
insanity defense. I was not the first person, nor will I be the last, to
find himself in opposition to some of the sacred principles of his
society and group. Lord Acton, for whom my admiration has grown
steadily through the years, had first-hand experience with this cir-
cumstance. Moreover, since he was a devoutly religious man, it must
have been harder for him to bear its ethical burden than it has been
for me. In his famous letter to his great mentor, Johann Joseph Ignaz
von Dollinger (1799-1890), Acton wrote:

> I came, very slowly and reluctantly indeed to the conclusion that they [the
> great Catholic notables] were dishonest. And I found out a special reason for
> their dishonesty in the desire to keep up the credit of authority in the Church...
> When I got to understand history from the sources, especially from unpub-
> lished sources, the reason of all this became obvious. There was a conspiracy
> to deceive... That men might believe the Pope, it was resolved to make them
> believe that vice is virtue and falsehood truth.[7]

Still, Acton prided himself that, "It takes a gentleman to live on
terms of hearty friendship and kindness and intimacy with men whose
ideas and conduct he abhors and when he well knows that they view

with contempt and horror the principles on which he shapes his own character and life."[8] As I look back on my life, I pride myself on having been able to follow Acton's example, at least in this regard.

I close with words I borrow from the immortal pen of Samuel Johnson (1709-1784). "I have protracted my work," he wrote in the preface to his *Dictionary*, "till most of those whom I wished to please, have sunk into the grave, and success and miscarriage are empty sounds; I therefore dismiss it with frigid tranquillity, having little to fear or hope from censure or from praise."[9]

Appendix I

The Power of False Truths:
The Maternity Hospital and the
Mental Hospital

Vague and insignificant forms of speech, and abuse of language, have for so long passed for mysteries of science; and hard and misapplied words, with little or no meaning, have, by prescription, such a right to be mistaken for deep learning and height of speculation, that it will not be easy to persuade either those who speak or those who hear them, that they are but the covers of ignorance, and hindrance of true knowledge.

—*John Locke (1690)*[1]

There is no error so monstrous that it fails to find defenders among the ablest men.

—*Lord Acton (1834-1902)*[2]

At first sight, the maternity hospital and the mental hospital seem two completely different institutions. However, on closer examination, striking similarities between them emerge. Both institutions appeared on the historical scene late in the seventeenth century, their creation signifying the change from an old religious to a new medical outlook on life. Both institutions were created to provide medical care for healthy persons, that is, for individuals not suffering from diseases.

Neither pregnancy nor delivery is a disease; each is an aspect of the mammalian reproductive mechanism. Women delivered babies long before special buildings called "lying-in hospitals" were established to care for them. Behavioral reactions to the vicissitudes of life are also not diseases; they are aspects of the repertoire of human actions. In the past, people who displayed such behaviors prospered or perished, were celebrated or condemned, long before there were special buildings called "mental hospitals," ostensibly devoted to their care.

In this Appendix, I comment on some important parallels between maternity hospitals and mental hospitals, especially the similarities between the iatrogenesis of *epidemic puerperal fever* and of *adult dependency as mental illness.*

The Lying-In Hospital and the Mental Hospital

Modern medicine begins in the middle of the nineteenth century, with the cellular theory of disease replacing the humoral theory of it.[3] The understanding of disease as a pathological alteration of cells, tissues, and organs was a *scientific achievement,* made possible in part by advances in technology, and in part by the establishment of municipal teaching hospitals that accommodated large numbers of patients. When the patients died, their corpses formed the "material" for the pathologist's postmortem examination. Rudolf Virchow, the "father" of scientific medicine, was a pathologist.

In England, hospitals began to be established more than a hundred years before the dawn of scientific medicine. These institutions resembled our current nursing homes and hospices more than they resemble our hospitals: they were de facto pre-burial sites, way-stations to the cemetery. Most of their would-be beneficiaries viewed entering them with the same dread with which people now view entering a nursing home. They were right. When persons of rank and wealth fell ill, they were cared for at home. And when it was time for them to die, they died at home. The aim of the early hospitals was social reform, not medical healing. Established as *philanthropic institutions,* their main aims were to relieve poor families of the burden of caring for sick relatives, provide pathologists with cadavers to advance the science of medicine, and furnish teachers and students of medicine "case material" for study and practice. Helping patients to recover from illness was an ancillary purpose, if that. When special lying-in hospitals were established, they were modeled after regular medical hospitals. Women from families with even modest means were rarely, if ever, delivered in maternity hospitals before the twentieth century.

The development of mental hospitals followed a similar pattern. The early private madhouses, established toward the end of the seventeenth century in England, were intended to help wealthy persons dispose of their unwanted relatives, by disguising the relative's coerced rehousing as care for insanity. However, after insane asylums became public institutions in the eighteenth century, their inmate population consisted almost entirely of paupers.

In hindsight, no medical historian doubts that, for the patients, the early hospitals, especially the maternity hospitals and madhouses, did more harm than good. Their real beneficiaries, as I noted, were not the patients, but rather the patients' families and the medical profession. In the case of mental hospitals, this is still the case, with the judicial system and lawyers as additional beneficiaries.

Prior to the twentieth century, hospitals were places of horror. However, the harm they could do was limited by the fact that most of the sick people who went there were hopelessly ill and would have soon died in any case. This, though, was not true for maternity hospitals and mental hospitals. The typical woman who entered a lying-in hospital was young and in excellent health. She would probably not have died had she delivered her infant at home, under seemingly unhygienic conditions. Her death was directly attributable to where she delivered, that is, the maternity hospital. Similarly, the typical person admitted to a mental hospital was a young adult in good health. Becoming a chronic mental patient was a direct consequence of being incarcerated for years in an insane asylum. Large public mental hospitals also housed people suffering from neurosyphilis and other fatal diseases of the nervous system. These patients, unlike the "mentally ill," soon died of their diseases.

Looking back at the history of lying-in hospitals, Irvine Loudon, an English medical historian, writes:

> Although intended to bring skill and comfort to the poor in childbirth, and save them from the perceived ignorance of untrained midwives, the lying-in hospitals were from the early years plagued by recurrent epidemics of puerperal fever with appalling mortality rates. By *choosing delivery* in a lying-in hospital, women (although they seldom knew it) were exposing themselves to a risk of dying that was many times higher than it would have been if they had stayed at home in the worst of slums and been attended in their birth by no one except family and an untrained midwife. The lying-in hospitals were such a disaster that, *in retrospect*, it would have been better if they had never been established before the introduction of antisepsis in the 1880s.[4]

Two points need to be made about Loudon's account. One is that women did not, as a rule, *choose* to be delivered in lying-in hospitals. Typically, they were dragged there by ignorant, overburdened relatives who wanted to be relieved of the duty of caring for them, and sometimes by public authorities imposing "enlightened medical care" on poor people helpless to resist their domination. The other point is that the detrimental nature of the lying-in hospital need not have been a retrospective judgment. It was obvious from the start, to many physicians as well as to many pregnant women. Repeatedly, conscientious physicians noted that outbreaks of puerperal fever often occurred only among women delivered by a particular midwife or physician, while women delivered by other attendants in the same area escaped the illness. After lying-in hospitals were built, physicians could not have helped but notice that puerperal fever occurred far more often among women delivered in such institutions than among women delivered in their homes.

Discovery of the Iatrogenesis of Puerperal Fever: A Brief History

Once a medical practice is officially accepted as "correct" and becomes the *standard of care*, it is very hard for doctors to resist it. To get along, you go along, and most physicians went along. During the first half of the nineteenth century, the medical profession, resting on new discoveries in chemistry and physics, began to acquire prestige and power it had not enjoyed in previous ages. Physicians claimed to have an explanation for virtually everything that ailed the human body. Puerperal fever was no exception: it was due to bad air, the so-called miasma theory. A few physicians dissented. In the United States, Oliver Wendell Holmes, and, in Austria-Hungary, Ignaz Semmelweis, declared publicly that puerperal fever was a contagious disease, transmitted to patients by the "dirty hands" of the doctors.

Actually, the contagious nature of puerperal fever was so obvious that it was widely recognized long before bacteria were discovered and their role in the pathogenesis of illness understood. However, in the absence of an understanding of the mechanism of contagion, the proponents of the infectious etiology of puerperal fever were in no position to overthrow the prevailing understanding of the disease, rendered persuasive and "true" by custom and medical authority. Moreover, the understanding of puerperal fever as a contagious-iatrogenic illness affronted and threatened the image of the physician as healer: the new explanation implicated the physician as the "cause" of the woman's illness and death. To sustain such a serious charge required that several elements come together: the precise mode of transmission and pathogenesis of puerperal fever had to be articulated and supported with irrefutable evidence; prestigious and powerful medical experts had to be willing to endorse it; and the powerful medical authorities who opposed the new theory had to grow old or die. In the case of puerperal fever, this process required almost a century.

As early as in 1795, the Scottish physician Alexander Gordon (1752-1799) published an account of epidemic puerperal fever in Aberdeen, stating: "I had evident proofs that every person who had been with a patient in the puerperal fever became charged with an atmosphere of infection which was communicated to every pregnant woman who happened to come within its sphere... *I myself was the means of carrying the infection to a great number of women...* These facts fully prove that the cause of the puerperal fever...[is] a specific contagion, or infection, altogether unconnected with a noxious condition of the atmosphere."[5]

In 1842, Oliver Wendell Holmes (1809-1894)—physician, professor of anatomy at Harvard Medical School, and later a celebrated author—published a pioneering paper, titled "The contagiousness of puerperal fever."[6] However, obstetrical authorities disdainfully dismissed this idea. Charles D. Meigs (1792-1869), professor of obstetrics at Jefferson Medical College in Philadelphia and the undisputed leader of the field in the United States, "was totally scornful of even the remote possibility of contagion... He dismissed the idea of a link between erysipelas and puerperal fever as rubbish. Erysipelas was a skin disease. How could you have erysipelas of the uterus? 'You might as well say that a woman has iritis of the pylorus, which would be absolute nonsense.'"[7]

About the same time, Ignaz Phillip Semmelweis (1818-1865), a Hungarian physician working at the large public hospital of the University of Vienna Medical School, began to observe that patients delivered by medical students and physicians developed puerperal fever much more often than did patients in the same hospital delivered by midwives. Semmelweis was unaware of Holmes's work. Like Holmes, he concluded that the physicians' hands carried an agent responsible for the disease. As if that were not bad enough, Semmelweis made another mistake: he proved it. "Beginning in May, 1847, Semmelweis made the medical students wash their hands with chlorinated lime water and, predictably, the mortality rates...dropped from 18.3% to 1.3%. So effective were his methods that *between March and August of 1848 no woman died in childbirth in that division.*"[8]

With this disturbing discovery, Semmelweis became living proof of the Hungarian proverb, "Tell the truth, and people will bash in your head." He was attacked for slandering the medical profession and his University teaching post was not renewed. "Returning to Hungary, Semmelweis repeated his successful attack on childbed fever at the St. Rochus Hospital in Pest [not yet united with Buda into the single city of Budapest], where he worked for the next six years, reducing the mortality rate to less than 1%."[9] For this, he got his head bashed in even more severely.[10]

Reviewing the history of puerperal fever, Gerald Weissmann, professor of medicine at New York University Medical Center, observes: "Although Semmelweis and Holmes were an ocean apart, their findings were complementary. Holmes had deduced contagion by his retrospective study of private practice and he advised relative asepsis as the remedy; Semmelweis studied contagion prospectively in a charity ward by testing antisepsis as the remedy. Holmes, unlike Semmelweis, lived to see his work accepted by his colleagues the world over."[11]

Only in the 1870s, after famed Scottish surgeon Joseph Lister (1827-1912) established antisepsis, did the correct understanding of puerperal fever become generally accepted in theory, and only then were the measures for preventing the disease, suggested by Semmelweis, adopted as correct obstetrical practice. Hailing Semmelweis as a martyr to puerperal fever, Lister declared: "Without Semmelweis, my achievements would be nothing."[12] This was hyperbole, a symptom, perhaps, of the medical profession's guilt for its mistreatment of this martyr to truth.

The Conflict Between Popular Opinion and Truth

The history of liberty, especially the liberty to denounce doctrine as delusion, is largely the story of the conflict between popular opinion as collective error and dissenting individual opinion as truth.[13] It does not follow, of course, that all rejection of popular opinion rests on an as-yet-undiscovered truth, although individuals with deviant ideas like to believe that opposition to their views is evidence of their validity. Especially where new truths threaten entrenched economic interests and established social habits, it usually takes a long time to sort out truth from error.

With the end of the nineteenth century, virtually all similarities between the maternity hospital and the mental hospital have ended.

Modern obstetrical units are a far cry from the maternity wards of Semmelweis' day. They are sanitary and, in case of complications, offer genuine life-saving treatments for both mother and newborn.

The medical utility of the modern maternity hospital *for the obstetrical patient* contrasts dramatically with the medical disutility of the modern mental hospital *for the mental patient*. Despite overwhelming evidence to the contrary, prominent psychiatrists, both in the United Kingdom and in the United States, continue to proclaim that there is no distinction between mental and physical illnesses, and therefore, by implication, none between medical and mental hospitals.[14] For example, in an editorial in the *British Journal of Psychiatry*, R. E. Kendell, professor of psychiatry at the University of Edinburgh, asserts that the distinction between mental and physical illness has "long been abandoned by all thinking physicians," and that "not only is the distinction between mental and physical illness ill-founded and incompatible with contemporary understanding of disease, it is also damaging to the long-term interests of patients themselves."[15] An editorial in the *British Journal of Medicine*, appearing at the same time as Kendell's, flatly contradicts his claims. Jennifer Leaning, professor of international health at Harvard Medical School, writes: "In 1986 and 1992 the BMA [British Medical Association] broke new ground in publishing reports on human rights *that documented what physicians were doing to the detriment of their patients...* The definition of human rights remained relatively restricted, however, in *concentrating on rights in closed institutions such as prisons and psychiatric hospitals.*"[16]

It is clear that as long as psychiatrists operate willingly and eagerly in a social milieu in which they have the duty and power to imprison so-called mental patients and "treat" them against their will, they are practicing psychiatric slavery. This interpretation is consistent with the uncontested fact, greatly troubling to psychiatrists, that many so-called psychiatric patients reject psychiatric services as harmful—not only at the time when they are subjected to such "help," but also in retrospect, when they look back at their lives many years after having been "patients."[17]

Some Personal Reminiscences and Reflections

I learned about Semmelweis as a child growing up in Budapest. I well remember the statue—Semmelweis standing and, at his feet, a mother, cradling an infant, gazing up at him adoringly—situated in a small park in front the St. Rochus Hospital, not far from the "Minta Gimnazium," the school I attended for the last eight years that Hungary was my home. I was deeply moved by the story of Semmelweis's tragic life. It taught me, at an early age, the lesson that it can be dangerous to be wrong, but, to be right, when society regards the majority's falsehood as truth, could be fatal. This principle is especially true with respect to "false truths" that form an important part of a whole society's belief system. In the past, such pivotal false truths were religious in nature. In the modern world, they are political and medical in nature. The lesson of Semmelweis's tragedy proved to be extremely helpful, virtually life-saving, for me.

Even as an adolescent, once I grasped the scientific concept of disease, it seemed to me obvious that many persons categorized as mentally ill and incarcerated in mental hospitals were not sick; instead, they exhibited behaviors unwanted by others, who diagnosed them as mad and locked them up; and that this is why, unlike medical patients, mental patients insist that they are not ill. In medical school, I began to understand clearly that my interpretation was correct—that mental illness is a myth. It is therefore foolish to look for the causes or cures of the imaginary ailments we call "mental diseases." *Diseases of the body* have causes, such as infectious agents or nutritional deficiencies; they can be prevented and cured by dealing with these causes. *Persons* said to have mental diseases, on the other hand, have reasons for their actions; reasons for such actions must be understood and represented the same way that novelists and playwrights understand and depict the motivations of fictional characters and their behaviors.

A deep sense of the invincible social power of false truths enabled me to conceal my ideas from representatives of received psychiatric wisdom until such time that I was no longer under their educational or economic control and could conduct myself in such a way that would minimize the chances of being cast in the role of "enemy of the people." Henrik Ibsen's famous play, *An Enemy of the People* (1882), is the dramatic story of a doctor whose work and fate are loosely modeled after the tragedy of Ignaz Semmelweis. Dr. Stockmann, a simple country doctor, tries to protect people from using the town bath contaminated with pathogenic bacteria. His discovery, however, conflicts with people's belief in the therapeutic properties of their treasured spa and jeopardizes their economic interests. The city's leaders and the public denounce Stockman as "an enemy of the people."

The waters Stockman denounced *had* to be therapeutic. Antipsychotic drugs *have* to be therapeutic, and schizophrenia *has* to be a brain disease. A *White House Fact Sheet on Myths and Facts about Mental Illness*, dated June 5, 1999, asserts that "Research in the last decade proves that mental illnesses are diagnosable disorders of the brain."[18] However, according to a report in the *British Medical Journal*, in May 2001, "Postmortem and imaging studies [of patients with schizophrenia] often fail to show the characteristic abnormalities of any known neurodegenerative disorders leading to the suspicion that a novel neuropathological process may be at large."[19]

This suggests two different inferences. One, entertained by the editors of the *British Medical Journal*, is "the suspicion that a novel neuropathological process may be at large." That suspicion forms the basis of psychiatry as a medical discipline and justifies psychiatric coercion as medical care.

The other inference is that there is no schizophrenia. That inference is so unpalatable—its implications are so devastating—that the authorities cannot deign to acknowledge it, even as a possibility. If there were no schizophrenia, there would be no medical, psychiatric, public health, or therapeutic justification for arresting, imprisoning, and involuntarily drugging people we call "schizophrenics." There would be no civil commitment and no insanity defense.

Where would that leave us?

Appendix II

Victims of Psychiatric Slavery: A Sampler

Homo homini lupus. (Man is wolf to man.)
—*Titus Maccius Plautus (c. 254 - c. 184 B.C.)[1]*

When you're told that...you are a madman or a criminal—that is, in short, when people suddenly turn their attention upon you—know, then, that you have fallen into a bewitched circle out of which you will nevermore escape. You will strive to escape—and will go still further astray. Yield, for no human exertion will any longer save you.
—*Anton Chekhov (1860-1904)[2]*

In 1970, in *The Manufacture of Madness*, I proposed the term "existential cannibalism" to describe the semantic-symbolic destruction of man by man, an activity that appears to be an essential part of social existence, especially in modern mass societies. I wrote: "Only through participating in the ritual destruction of the Other, only through committing existential cannibalism, is man admitted to membership in the modern State... The cannibal incorporates his victim to give himself virtue; we expel ours to give ourselves innocence... To refuse to persecute the socially accredited scapegoat is interpreted as an attack on society itself."[3]

Human beings may be divided into two groups: one comprises persons who participate in the drama of existential cannibalism, as predators or preys, the other of persons who refuse to play either role. Most people—especially psychiatrists and mental patients—fall into the first group. Men such as Voltaire, Acton, and Mencken exemplify persons who fall into the second group.

As long as mental health professionals have the authority and duty to exercise legally authorized force over others and do so, they are predators—existential cannibals who cast their victims into what

Chekhov aptly called "a bewitched circle," out of which there is no escape. Reciprocally, persons who seek mental health services or so conduct themselves as to invite the attention of mental health professionals are prey—existential fodder in society's ceaseless war on scapegoated deviants.

Having long considered psychiatry as similar to slavery, in 1973 I published an anthology, titled *The Age of Madness*, composed partly of the autobiographical writings of the victims of psychiatric slavery, and partly of pieces critical of psychiatric coercion written by well-known men of letters.[4] This Appendix may be considered an addendum to that anthology.

I begin with a little-known piece by John Stuart Mill, a letter to a newspaper editor written in 1858, protesting the domination of the mental patient by the psychiatrist. It illustrates how, despite often-touted scientific advances in psychiatry, with respect to the practice of involuntary mental hospitalization, very little has changed during the past 150 years.

The other vignettes are all from recent sources. They offer the reader a direct view, unencumbered by commentary, of contemporary psychiatric practices, often falsely characterized as psychiatric abuses. I say "falsely characterized" because I regard all psychiatric practices that rely on force and fraud—instead of contract and cooperation—as psychiatric abuses.

*   *   *

The Law of Lunacy, by John Stuart Mill *(Daily News,* London, 1858)

It has become urgently necessary that public attention should be called to the state of the law on the subject of Lunacy, and the frightful facility with which any persons whom their heirs or connexions desire to put out of the way, may be consigned without trial to a fate more cruel and hopeless than the most rigorous imprisonment.

Recent circumstances have made it a matter of notoriety, that confinement in a madhouse is the wisest means of getting rid of, or bringing to terms, refractory wives... A perfectly innocent person can be fraudulently kidnapped, seized, and carried off to a madhouse on the assertion of any two so-called medical men, who have scarcely seen the victim whom they dismiss to a condition far worse than penalty which the law inflicts for proved crime. Convicts are not delivered over to the absolute power of their gaoler; nor can they be subjected to the ruffianly treatment revealed by the York inquiry. Convicts can appeal against ill treatment; but to other unfortunates the ordinary use of speech is virtually denied; their somber statements of facts, still more their passionate protests against injustice, are held to be so many instances of insane delusion...

The obvious remedy is to require the same guarantees before depriving a fellow-creature of liberty on one pretext as on another... Many other improvements in the law and procedure in these cases are urgently needed... I earnestly entreat you to continue your efforts at rousing public opinion on a matter so vital to the freedom and security of the subject.[5]

Not Guilty by Reason of Insanity *(Newsday, August 2001)*

October 8, 1981, Tommy Coberg and three other teenagers were arrested in the attempted robbery of a 13-year-old. The three others, then 15, appeared in Family Court, and their records remain sealed. But Coberg had just turned 17, just old enough to face criminal prosecution. His lawyer advised his parents that he should plead not guilty by reason of mental defect, or insanity—a strategy he said would avoid a 1-year prison sentence and lifelong criminal record. With the plea, the lawyer said, Coberg could expect to spend a few months in a children's psychiatric facility.

Coberg took the advice, and the lawyer told the court that he suffered from borderline mental retardation and didn't understand the consequences of his actions when he participated in the crime. But instead of spending a short time in a children's facility, Coberg wound up spending almost all of the next 20 years locked inside the state's mental health system.

Four months ago he walked out of the Pilgrim State Psychiatric Center in Brentwood into "conditional" freedom. He is 36 years old. For the next five years, Coberg must adhere to terms of his release: Live in a group home until he successfully petitions to live on his own; stay in New York State; and keep out of trouble. Only then, he says, will he know what it is to be truly free. "I want my life back," says Coberg, a small-framed man with a boyish smile. "I still can't believe what happened to my life..."

Doctors initially gave Coberg a diagnosis: antisocial personality disorder, a diagnosis generally saved for adults with criminal backgrounds. The diagnosis persisted—along with two other behavioral diagnoses—through the years. It wasn't until 1997 that a mix of doctors, lawyers and friends came together to fight their own battle for Coberg. They finally won this year. Doctors, lawyers and hospital officials now say that Coberg is no longer mentally ill or a danger to himself or others. Many of those involved in Coberg's case say it's hard to know if that diagnosis was ever appropriate.

Last year, during a hearing to determine whether Coberg's patient privileges should be extended, Pilgrim's associate medical director testified: "I think this fellow is being shortchanged in his treatment. What I found was, in talking to staff at all different levels, is a lot of people just didn't like Tommy," Dr. Michael Slome testified...

Defendants who dispose of the charges against them by entering an insanity plea often spend considerably more time in psychiatric hospitals than they would have in jail. According to Henry Steadman, a sociologist at Policy Research Associates in Delmar, N.Y., defendants in New York State who plead not guilty by reason of insanity to violent crimes serve twice as long in the mental health system as defendants convicted of comparable offenses. When the crimes are nonviolent, the insanity defendants serve four times as long—even longer, according to other studies...

In one study, Steadman said he analyzed the reasons insanity "acquitees" were hospitalized in eight states and found 50 percent of them were being detained for nonviolent crimes. Even though these studies were conducted in the 1980s, things haven't gotten better, Steadman said. "This is unethical behavior on the part of attorneys who plead [their clients] not guilty by reason of insanity for misdemeanor crimes..."

Coberg's story illustrates what some mental health experts say is a flaw in the insanity defense. "Once you're in the [mental health] system, it doesn't matter whether you've murdered someone or stolen a candy bar," said Sid Hirschfeld, director of the Mental Hygiene Legal Service, a state-funded legal advocacy organization that represents mental patients in the New York State in-patient system. "It's up to the patient to figure out how to get out..."

The prosecutor who argued to keep Coberg institutionalized disputes the notion that his psychiatric sentence was too harsh. "These cases are tough," said Guy Arcidiacono, deputy chief of the forensic unit for the Suffolk County district attorney's office. "Tom's been his worst enemy... The fact that he was in so long demonstrates that he really needs treatment," he said. "To my mind, the system really worked."

Brooks and other mental-health experts disagree and contend the insanity defense puts patients at a disadvantage. They become so-called CPL-330.20 patients, characterized for a section of the Criminal Procedure Law that says the "burden is on the patients to prove that they are not dangerous and will never be again," Brooks said. "Patients get the short end of the stick. "Clinicians will spend years justifying that decision," Brooks said...

Coberg's diagnosis has been altered over the years: From poor impulse control to antisocial personality disorder to intermittent explosive disorder. Psychiatrists recently hired to review his case said they believe the stress of being locked away contributed to his aggression. "He's not crazy," said Richard L. Weidenbacher Jr., a psychiatrist who has known Coberg for about five years and was one of those recently advocating for his release. "It's high time to get him out...he's been hospitalized so long that it has rendered him incapable of taking responsibility for his actions." Weidenbacher and others agree that Coberg never had a chance to grow up and learn appropriate adult behavior. "That is the very reason I want him out [of the system]. He has to learn to take responsibility for his conduct... He's not mentally ill or dangerous..." During most of the past two decades, Coberg received no medical treatment for a severe psychiatric disorder, Weidenbacher said...

Coberg had just celebrated his 17th birthday a month earlier and, upon his arrest, was charged as an adult with second-degree attempted robbery. His parents did not post the $150 bail. They hired Barry Warren to defend their son, and the family agreed with the recommendation to enter the insanity plea. In 1985, his behavior had been good enough for psychiatrists to release him. But within a year, a fight erupted between Coberg and his mother, Arlene, and she called the police, telling them her son had picked up a knife in a threatening way. He was returned to the mental health system. In 1998, Coberg's brother Joseph wrote to the courts describing the events of that day: "My mother picked up the knife and threatened Thomas..."

Michael Welner, a forensic psychiatrist in New York, said attorneys, prosecutors, administrators and "acquitees" have come to recognize an unwritten rule: "The insanity acquitee must prove, beyond a reasonable doubt, that he will never again break the law. It is a system that offers hope, then pulls it away, and then expects

acquitees to tolerate frustration as a sign of clinical improvement—
a standard not even expected of prison inmates..."

"Will I ever have a chance at a normal life?" he [Coberg] asked.
"There were so many times I just said, 'God, give me jail. At least I'd
know I would get out...'"

The other teenagers involved in the attempted robbery 20 years
ago have all had a chance to move on. "Nothing ever happened to
any of us," said Paul, who, when contacted by *Newsday*, asked that
his last name not be used. He is a house-painter. "That kid serving 20
years is unjust," said Paul. "It's scary. It's like saying someone got
charged with murder and 20 years later they found the real killer...⁶

Mental Illness by Mandate (*Los Angeles Times*, February 2000)

In 1950s Quebec, the Catholic Church turned orphanages into
psychiatric hospitals overnight—purely for economic reasons. To
the now-middle-aged victims, it amounted to nothing less than selling their souls.

Herve Bertrand remembers the day when his life at a Quebec orphanage turned inside out. "On March 18, 1954, the nuns came in
and said, 'From today, you are all crazy.' Everyone started to cry,
even the nuns. Then everything changed: Our lessons stopped, and
work—they called it therapy—began. I saw the bars go on the win-
dows, the fences go up around the compound. I saw the autobuses
pull up full of psychiatric patients—our new roommates. It was like
a prison. And that's where I spent a quarter of my life."

Bertrand, 57, was among more than 3,000 children living in 12
Quebec orphanages that the Roman Catholic Church transformed—
some virtually overnight—into mental hospitals in the 1940s and
'50s to reap more generous government subsidies. A policy ordained
by Quebec's then-premier, Maurice Duplessis, granted the institutions more than three times the amount of money to care for a mental patient than they received for orphans. So, in order that the children would qualify, their medical records were altered to declare
them mentally unstable or retarded.

But that was not just a change of labels, say the now-middle-aged
orphans: The church sold their souls. Many were treated like mental
patients, with unnecessary drugs and straightjackets. It took the orphans nearly 40 years to organize and ask the church and state for
redress. They finally got an answer last year. Quebec Premier Lucien
Bouchard apologized for his predecessor's mistakes and offered

nominal compensation. But he also praised the "great deal of devotion" of the nuns who cared for the children.

Church officials were less contrite. "They don't deserve an apology," said Cardinal Jean-Claude Turcotte, adding that real responsibility lay not with the religious community, but with the parents for their wayward lifestyles. While the government and the church resist confronting the past, members of this damaged generation are still trying to find closure and compensation for the childhood they will never recover...

Not all the children were orphans. Many, like Bertrand, had been born out of wedlock and were viewed by the church as children of sin. Others came from families too poor to care for them who were urged to put them in the hands of nuns for a proper religious upbringing. But the sisters were overwhelmed—a single nun was typically in charge of 50 children, say people who were familiar with the institutions at the time. They were women with no child-rearing experience, undertrained and overworked. They transferred their culture of penitence and self-discipline to children who didn't understand. In an institutional setting, this could quickly turn into abuse, and few of the children had family visitors who could intervene.

St.-Julien Hospital was one of the earliest psychiatric institutions to take orphans, starting in the 1940s. Alice Quinton, 62, was born of an incestuous relationship and transferred to St.-Julien from an orphanage in 1945. On her admission form, the reason for her entry is written in a nun's precise cursive: "Cause of scandal." That year, when Quinton was 7, the nuns told Alice that her parents were dead, and in turn reported to her mother that Alice had died. And in a way, Quinton says, she did die that year. Her childhood, spent amid 500 other orphans and 900 mentally ill adults, is a dark memory of cells, tranquilizers and straitjackets. She says she was punished for asking questions, for wetting her bed, for not doing her work fast enough.

"I asked, 'Why am I here?' No one ever had an answer. I thought to myself: 'Am I going crazy? Am I going to grow up to be like these mental patients?'" Today, Quinton carries a binder of grievances, a catalog of injustice. She opens it to show an architectural diagram of St.-Julien, featuring the layout of her ward and the location of the bed where she says she was strapped in a straitjacket on the cold metal springs for three weeks... "None of it made sense," she says, her eyes brimming. "But I never thought I was insane. I never believed I was retarded."

In the summer of 1960, a Montreal psychiatric team began a series of investigations that would prove her right. At one of the institutions, Mont Providence, an examination of about 500 boys and girls aged 4 through 12 revealed that most were of normal intelligence but being impaired by institutionalization. "One of the conclusions of the report was that many children were perfectly intelligent but perfectly ignorant," says Dr. Jean Gaudreau, one of six doctors who evaluated the children. "In one of the tests, we showed the children objects—keys, a flag, a stove, a refrigerator. Many of the children couldn't name them, not because of a lack of intelligence but because they had never seen one." Gaudreau, now a psychology professor at the University of Montreal, recalls his shock at the pervasive stench of urine, at seeing a 5-year-old boy in a straitjacket, tied to a drainpipe, and teenagers drugged with tranquilizers. "Most of them were not retarded when they went in," he says. "Some of them were by the time they got out."

That investigation was the beginning of the end of the program. After psychiatrist Denis Lazure headed a wider investigation in 1962, inspecting 15 of the province's hospitals, a new government declared that the children did not belong in institutions and released them that year. The younger ones went to other orphanages or foster homes. The older ones were on their own. "Contrary to the popular belief of some, there is no exaggeration in the accounts of the sufferings of the Duplessis orphans," says Lazure, who became the Quebec health minister after the study. "If anything, they've been understated..."

Bertrand, now a plumber, is frustrated by the religious orders' denials, then and now. He describes repeated sexual abuse: When the nuns went to church, a guard would come and get him, strap him in a straitjacket and sodomize him. "I told the nuns," he says, "but they didn't believe me." His hospital records from Mont Providence describe rectal damage so severe that surgery was recommended.

Even today, nuns who ran the orphanages refuse to comment on what happened in that era. Last February, Cardinal Turcotte, a senior representative of the Catholic Church in Canada, said, "I wholeheartedly defend the devoted religious women who gave 40 to 50 years of their lives working in the institutions." Turcotte called the orphans "victims of life," and declared, "They don't deserve an apology."

While some Quebeckers agree that the issue is nearly half a century old and should be left behind, Bertrand emphasizes that the orphans' entire lives, not just their childhoods, were affected. When his children were born, he says, he re-encountered the shadows of his youth. "I was not a good father. I was too aggressive. I slapped the children because I did not know how to discipline them kindly. I thought I could leave the past behind, but I still have all that in my head."

Bruno Roy, 56, who was in Mont Providence with Bertrand, is one who has reclaimed his life. Born out of wedlock, he lived in another orphanage until he was transferred to Mont Providence at age 7. Before the institution converted to a psychiatric facility, his medical chart read: "This child demonstrates normal intelligence and is capable of being educated—he is fairly well adapted and has achieved the emotional maturity of children his age." After Mont Providence's status changed, his record declared him "severely mentally retarded."

Today, Roy has a doctorate in French literature and teaches at a Quebec college. A burly man whose black beard is stippled with gray, he has written 12 books on poetry and literature—and one about his childhood experiences that brought attention to the whole issue. "Yes, it's true. I'm a mental defective," he says, leaning back in a chair and laughing. Roy has become an effective spokesman for the rest of the orphans, many of whom he describes matter-of-factly as "damaged goods."

He was saved, he says, by one kind nun who recognized his spark and put him in a vocational training program when he was 15, just to get him outside the compound's walls. He worked in a cardboard box factory and tried to make up for lost time. He realized he had no vocabulary for the outside world. "In the years inside Mont Providence, I saw the violence and absurdity, yet I didn't see it, because to me it was normal. I didn't have anything to compare it to," he says. At first, he says, it was easier to bury his experience. For 30 years, while he became a successful scholar, he did not talk about his past. "Then one day, one of my [Mont Providence] classmates called and said: 'You made it, but we're still less than human. Won't you help defend us?'

"I went to a meeting and saw the faces of people who were totally destroyed. These were my old playmates, who were normal when we were kids. Now they are broken. They had no voice. They had no credibility. No one would believe their horrible stories." In 1994 he wrote a book, "My Memories From the Asylum," to document what had happened to them all. "I became a writer because of one sentence by our national poet, Gaston Miron: 'One day I will have said yes to my birth.'" It was a turning point not only for Roy but for other Duplessis orphans. But though their case began to receive national attention, justice continued to elude them.

A class-action lawsuit was rejected by a provincial court in 1995 on the grounds that it would be too difficult to determine individual damages in the hundreds of different cases. Later that year, a police investigation of 321 complaints, including Bertrand's accusation of rape backed up by medical documents, concluded that the evidence of abuse was too old and unreliable. So in 1997, the Duplessis orphans tried a different tactic. They formed a committee to ask for a public inquiry, plus compensation and apologies from the church and government... The government assigned an ombudsman, Daniel Jacoby, to examine the matter...

Last March, Premier Bouchard did apologize on behalf of the Quebec government and offered a fund equivalent to $2.1 million to provide social services for the orphans who need them—about $700 total per victim. But the offer included no direct compensation for individuals or acknowledgment of pain and suffering. The orphans' committee declared it an insult...

Msgr. Pierre Morissette, head of the Assembly of Quebec Bishops, told a news conference in September that an apology by the church "would betray the work of those who dedicated their lives to the poorest in society." A spokeswoman for the assembly, Rolande Parrot, said in a December interview that the church does not take any responsibility for the transfer of children to psychiatric hospitals and does not consider the religious community to have done anything wrong. She dismissed the orphans committee's protests and its vows that it will pursue the matter all the way to the Vatican. "There are no plans to reopen the case," Parrot said.[7]

[Addendum: In July 2002, about 1,000 of the orphans who were wrongfully moved to mental institutions have accepted a settlement compensation offer from Quebec province for $16.7 million, or about $16,650 each.[8] None of the numerous accounts of this story on the Internet faults psychiatrists or psychiatry. None compares the Canadian psychiatrists' crimes against orphans to the Nazi psychiatrists' crimes against crippled children and mental patients. Not accused of wrongdoing, the psychiatrists do not apologize for wrongdoing. T. S.]

Psychiatry in Israel (*Ha'aretz*, November 9, 2000)

Mentally ill patients committed to hospitals in Israel are held in worse conditions than prisoners, Tel Aviv District Court Judge Saviona Rotlevy charged in a decision handed down earlier this week... The judge ordered the release of a woman who had been committed to a closed ward in Abarbanel Hospital in Bat Yam. Rotlevy ruled that her forced hospitalization was unjustified, and that it involved a series of illegal proceedings carried out by senior psychiatrists at the Ministry of Health and attorneys in the State Prosecutor's Office. The ruling marked the first time that an Israeli judge has referred to commitment to mental institutions as "imprisonment" and not just "hospitalization." The Ministry of Health has lobbied against the use of the term "imprisonment" to refer to forced hospitalization of mentally ill patients.

The patient, a 50-year-old resident of northern Israel, was committed to the mental hospital in September upon the request of her son. The hospitalization order was issued by the ministry's deputy psychiatrist in the Tel Aviv region, Dr. Uzi Shai, and the psychiatrist of the Haifa region, Dr. Danny Enoch... The patient's attorney, Ilan Yacobovich, told the court that the doctors handling her case had placed themselves "above the law" and that "time after time" the psychiatrists had committed "blatant and systematic violations of the law." He argued that the regional psychiatrists in Haifa and Tel Aviv had demonstrated "the miserable status of mental patients' rights in Israel...not a phenomenon that pertains to only one region..."

Judge Rotlevy continued: "It gives one goosebumps to read the material in the medical file. How is it possible that today, in the 21st century, after the legislation of basic laws, and after nearly 10 years have passed since the law was amended to prevent the unnecessary commitment of mental patients, that the various authorities are still ignoring the law's directives and court rulings, and continue to do whatever they wish regarding the forced hospitalization of citizens?" The judge noted that "the patient was defined as posing an immediate physical danger to herself and her surroundings without this ever being suitably explained... There is indeed a story of slapping her grown son, but even if this fact were true, it's hard to believe that in the year 2000 this would provide a basis for determining that a person poses physical and immediate dangers to her surroundings, and that this would justify her forced hospitalization. The situation of forcibly hospitalized mental patients is more difficult than prisoners, not only because they did not commit any crimes, but because their dignity is taken from them through medication that often leaves them without the ability to speak, think, express and react," the judge wrote.[9]

A "Crazy" Hungarian Prisoner of War (*The Times*, London, August 25, 2000)

Memories of home and war are flooding back for Andras Tamas, who has returned to his native Hungary after more than half a century in isolation in a Russian psychiatric hospital... Mr. Tamas is about 75. No one knows for sure. He remembers little of his five decades as a prisoner of war deep in northern Russia... Diagnosed by his captors as psychotic, after the war he was shunted through a series of Soviet prison camps to a psychiatric hospital 300 miles east of Moscow. There he lived for 53 years, never learning Russian, until rescued two weeks ago from lonely old age by a series of coincidences. The changes in his life since then are scarcely imaginable. For the first time since 1945 he is enjoying conversation, writing, and reading newspapers, experiences that have peeled away a shell of deep introspection, revealing words and phrases from a bygone age...

Tamas's first glimmer of hope came in 1992, when a local policeman of Slovak origin who often visited the hospital realized that the lonely patient spoke Hungarian. Years later, a local newspaper article about him was picked up by a Hungarian television bureau in Moscow... Since his return to Hungary he has not mentioned Kotelnich or Russia once but he has been deluged with invitations and gifts of money. He is owed £17,000 in army pension arrears and will soon be well—and rich—enough to buy a small house, where he is expected to live with minimal supervision.[10]

[On September 7, 2000, the story about Tamas appeared in the *Chicago Tribune*.]

...A month ago, a bewildered Tamas returned to a hero's welcome at the Budapest airport. The local press dubbed him "the last prisoner of World War II." Journalists told the incredible story of a young Hungarian conscript wrongly committed to a Russian mental institution and kept there because Russian authorities, failing to recognize his words as Hungarian, thought he was speaking gibberish... Records indicate the Russian doctors knew he was a Hungarian-speaking POW and that they diagnosed him as a schizophrenic. "The Russian documentation is very exact," said Veer [Andras Veer, head of the Hungarian National Institute of Psychiatry and Neurology], who has traveled to Kotelnich and examined the handwritten records. "It appears he was well-diagnosed and that he received valid psychiatric treatment. You have to remember that this was the late 1940s. This illness could not have been treated more successfully someplace else, not in Paris, not in Vienna, not in the United States," he said...

Little news from the outside world penetrated the walls of Kotelnich. Whatever books or newspapers may have been available, Tamas couldn't have read anyway. For a time, he attempted to write in Hungarian, but hospital authorities, suspicious of anything written in a language they couldn't understand, put a stop to that. With no one to speak to in his native language, his command of Hungarian began to wither... His plight was not discovered until the late 1990s when he was taken to a general hospital to be treated for high blood pressure and circulatory problems. There he had a chance encounter with a Russian doctor of Slovak origin who recognized Tamas' words as Hungarian... [11]

[Andras Veer, the head of the Hungarian National Institute of Psychiatry and Neurology, defends his Russian colleagues: "It appears he (Tamas) was well-diagnosed and that he received valid psychiatric treatment." T. S.]

Mental Health Care in Ghana (*The Lancet*, 2001)

There are currently just 13 psychiatrists for Ghana's population of 18 million people. The doctors' efforts to provide a service under such circumstances is admirable. But, within the state psychiatric system, there are also problems with policy and management... As a result some psychiatric provision is extremely negative, violating patients' rights and safety.

Although, legally, patients may be "voluntary," in practice they may be prevented from leaving. Some patients are locked in hospital for years without assessment. Some are "vagrants" brought in by the police.

An extreme example of this inhuman treatment is seen at the "special ward" of Accra Psychiatric Hospital, where about 300 men are locked in a set of cells designed for 50... [These] patients have no access to the outside world or to therapeutic help. Associate professor of psychiatry at the hospital, Samuel Turkson, confirmed patients' allegations of abuse. "Beatings with sticks are still used. Medication is used as punishment... Turkson estimates that half of the "voluntary" patients have no recognizable mental health problem...

Samuel Ohene, a lecturer at the University of Ghana's psychiatry department and a consultant psychiatrist as the Accra Psychiatric Hospital, said: "I have seen somebody who is blind from some chemical being put in their eyes, probably because he was having visual hallucinations. Or something is dropped in the ears to stop voices and auditory hallucinations...[12]

Testing the Faith: Student Sues College for Psychiatric Abuse, Sent to Mental Ward After He Objected to Play Depicting Jesus as Homosexual (*WorldNetDaily.com*, 2001)

A junior at Temple University in Philadelphia, Pa., is suing university officials for allegedly having him involuntarily committed to a psychiatric ward following a dispute over a play depicting Jesus Christ as a homosexual.

According to Brian Fahling, an attorney with the AFA Law Center in Tupelo, Miss., which is handling the case, Michael A. Marcavage was detained after he "initiated a Christian response" to the university theater department's decision to stage "Corpus Christi," a play that made its debut on Broadway in 1998 and depicts Jesus as a homosexual who has sex with his disciples.

In the play, Jesus was eventually crucified for being "king of the queers." When it broke on Broadway, the play received national criticism.

Marcavage, a former White House West Wing intern, immediately complained about the play to the dean of the School of Communications and Theater, as well as the president of the university—whom Fahling said has since left Temple—when theater officials announced it in the fall of 1999.

Besides informing those officials of the play's content, Fahling said Marcavage—in a prepared statement—admitted posting fliers all over the university "so that all Christians on campus would be aware of this horrible play," and made plans to stage a protest outside the theater when the play opened.

In the days that followed, Marcavage said he had a number of meetings with William Bergman, vice president of campus safety, and Carl Bittenbender, director of campus safety. Though he had initially planned to protest, Bergman and Bittenbender eventually convinced Marcavage that protests might lead to confrontations between rival student factions. Marcavage then agreed to cancel his protest. Instead, he asked officials for permission to stage a Christian outreach to students; Fahling said the university security officials gave him permission for that.

Marcavage, in his statement to Fahling, said Bergman promised him a stage would be provided to help him with his outreach program, but later the same day, Bittenbender allegedly called Marcavage to tell him that the stage "might be out of the question." The campus safety director then asked the student to meet with him and Bergman the next morning at the vice president's office.

At that meeting, Marcavage said Bergman told him a stage would be too expensive to provide and therefore, one would not be set up for the outreach program. Marcavage said he then offered to pay for the stage himself, but was again told no—without further explanation.

Exasperated, Marcavage said he then "excused himself, went to the bathroom, locked the door and prayed about what he should do next," AFA officials said.

According to the student, Bergman followed him to the bathroom and began pounding on the door, demanding that he open it and resume the discussion about the stage. Marcavage said he opened the door and "told him that I believed our conversation was over."

Next, according to Marcavage, Bergman "physically" forced him back into the vice president's office and "pushed me into a chair and held me with his arm." Fahling said Marcavage asked to leave but Bergman "allegedly refused to allow it."

"Attempting to rise, [Marcavage] said the vice president tripped him to the floor," then was "manhandled" to a nearby couch by both men "where they held him down."

Within moments, Marcavage said, a Temple University police officer arrived and handcuffed him. Then, "Marcavage was taken by police...to the Emergency Crisis Center at Temple University Hospital," AFA officials told WorldNetDaily.

According to Fahling, under Pennsylvania law, a person that is involuntarily committed for a psychological evaluation "has to be a clear threat to himself or a clear threat to others," though he and Marcavage deny that the student "in any way" fits the criteria.

Fahling said on-site interviews at the university with fellow students who personally know Marcavage—including one who is a registered nurse and saw him that morning before his meeting with officials—"indicated that he is not the kind of person" who would engage in behavior requiring a mandatory mental examination.

Yet, at the crisis center, Bittenbender allegedly signed a statement describing Marcavage as "severely mentally disabled"; that he represented a "clear and present danger to others"; that he had "inflicted or attempted to inflict serious bodily harm on another" within the past month; and that he "has attempted suicide"—all of which constituted a "reasonable probability of suicide unless treatment was afforded" him.

Fahling said Bittenbender concluded his statement by asserting that Marcavage was "in need of involuntary examination and treatment."

"When I was first told about this case, I found it hard to believe," Fahling told WorldNetDaily. "I thought it was something out of the 'Twilight Zone.'"

He said that Marcavage was not found to be mentally distressed or exhibiting any behavior that matched the admission statement given by Bittenbender. "He was released three hours later—and that was largely because it took [hospital staff] a while to get to him."

Fahling said Dr. Jose Villaluz of the clinic staff did examine Marcavage "because, per state law, they are required to. But he didn't find anything wrong with him."

The AFA attorney said documents provided by Marcavage show that Villaluz noted in his evaluation report that the student was "not in need of involuntary treatment."

Fahling added that when Marcavage was being led out of Bergman's office by police, a university staff psychologist—Dr. Denise Walton—was on hand and commented that she couldn't understand why the student was being involuntarily detained.

In a separate statement, Fahling said Walton wrote that she had seen "no overt sign that [Marcavage] was about to harm himself or others."

"This is a young man of some substance," Fahling said. "I believe his story is genuine. This kid is solid as a rock."

After being released, Marcavage said he tried to file a complaint with the university police department, but was rebuffed and told officers could not take a complaint against Bergman because he "is our boss."

While still at the police station, Bergman arrived and allegedly told Marcavage that no report would be filed "because no crime had been committed," the AFA Law Center said.

"His only recourse was to file a report with the Philadelphia Police Department," said the center, but it was unclear if Marcavage made that attempt.

However, the student did try to complain through other university channels, but after those also failed, he made the decision to contact the law center and file suit.

"Besides being a college student on the Dean's List, Michael was a White House intern with security clearance, is founder and president of a ministry called Protect the Children, president of his own business, and a volunteer who has worked with Campus Crusade for Christ and gone overseas with Feed the Children," Fahling said.

"This is a good Christian kid who wanted to stand up for Jesus, and instead was handcuffed and dragged to a mental hospital as if he'd been seeing pink elephants," he added.

Efforts to contact the university were unsuccessful.

Fahling did not disclose the amount of settlement Marcavage is seeking. He said Bergman and Bittenbender are named as co-defendants in the suit.[13]

The Cuckoo's Nest Revisited (*The Washington Post*, December 17, 2001)

Dozens of mentally ill men and women in Virginia have spent years locked up in state mental institutions for offenses as minor as breaking a window, spitting, indecent exposure and trespassing. They landed in maximum-security psychiatric wards—where they cannot step outside without an escort—after pleading not guilty by reason of insanity to misdemeanors committed during mental breakdowns or periods when they had stopped taking medication. But under Virginia's criminal justice system, which for a decade has emphasized public safety in cases involving the mentally ill, those acquitted of crimes because of mental illness have languished in hospitals that function as jails. Some have been there 10 years or more. Peeping Toms and people who cursed at police officers share wards with rapists and killers.

Now, prodded by advocates for the mentally ill, a bipartisan commission of state lawmakers is recommending legislation that would limit how long a nonviolent offender can be locked up. About 250 men and women are in state mental institutions because of crimes. As of last week, state officials say, 40 had committed misdemeanors, crimes that otherwise would carry jail sentences of no more than a year. State law allows them to be held in the treatment centers indefinitely.

The charges include public drunkenness, unwanted touching, slapping, cursing and petty larceny by a homeless person who stole for survival. The average stay is three years, officials said, though some people have been confined for six or more years. One man charged with breaking a window has been held in Central State Hospital outside Petersburg for 13 years, the report says. Some influential lawmakers describe the system as woefully broken. "I have great concern about us keeping somebody incarcerated or detained for 12 years for insignificant offenses," said Sen. Kenneth W. Stolle (R-Virginia Beach), a former police officer who heads the Virginia State Crime Commission and is a key lawmaker on criminal justice issues. "Most legislators would be surprised and shocked to find out somebody arrested for a misdemeanor has spent 12 years in jail when they could have spent a maximum of one year," Stolle said.

A 50-page report strongly critical of the policy is scheduled for release by the commission tomorrow. The insanity defense has left many people confined in institutions for the criminally insane indefinitely under a system that is "excessively hesitant" to release them, the report says. "For those charged with misdemeanors, particularly nonviolent misdemeanors, there may be little or no justification at all for extended confinement," it says. State mental health officials said they have tried to weigh public safety concerns against the individual freedoms of patients. Some patients who land in the system on minor charges have violent histories and could pose a danger to themselves or others, said James Morris, director of forensic services for the Virginia Department of Mental Health, Mental Retardation and Substance Abuse Services.

But Morris acknowledged that some nonviolent people could be released and said his agency is trying to make the system for evaluating patients more efficient. "Nobody should be criminalized for being mentally ill," he said. "We're looking to have the most humanitarian approach." Although patients can petition for release annually for five years, "the standards used and the lack of a burden placed on the government to demonstrate why confinement must continue" render the hearings "nothing more than ineffective formalities," the report says. After five years, patients can ask the court for release only every other year. Had they simply pleaded guilty in court, they would have been released on probation or served brief sentences. Defense lawyers say that paradox creates an ethical quandary for them. "If you know your client may be held within the mental health system for years on a traffic charge, is it proper to pursue an insanity defense?" asked Fairfax County defense lawyer Peter Greenspun. "It is not necessarily in their best interest to avoid a conviction."

Because of these issues, Virginia spends millions of dollars a year to care for people already suffering from scarce resources in their communities. With dozens of patients confined long-term for petty crimes—at an annual cost of $160,000 per bed—acutely ill patients who need hospital treatment sometimes are turned away, advocates say. The situation has created another danger, the report says. Seriously ill patients who need care sometimes plead guilty to save themselves from lengthy confinement and serve only brief jail time, if any. They are released without treatment, increasing the chances that they will commit other crimes.

The calls for reform are the latest troubles for a system with a history of poor treatment, patient deaths and abuses, and a handful of investigations by the U.S. Department of Justice. The government ended its four-year investigation of Central State in October, saying the hospital had improved conditions and its level of treatment.

Raymond Denk's crime was spitting on Prince William County sheriff's deputies outside a Haymarket restaurant in 1997. The officers had been trying to serve a detention order that would have committed him to a mental hospital for evaluation. On the advice of his attorney, Denk, who has manic depression, pleaded insanity and was committed to Central State. After three months, he was transferred to Northern Virginia Mental Health Institute, a 127-bed hospital in Falls Church. There he had more freedom, and he says his illness was treated. But it was nearly two years before a Manassas judge, agreeing with his doctors, set Denk free and said he no longer posed a risk to himself or others.

The decision came over the objections of a forensic review panel that said he had not completed a gradual process of receiving more privileges to show how well he could behave.

Denk, a divorced father of three, acknowledges a history of substance abuse and said he has been hospitalized periodically for the last 20 years. He is now back in the Northern Virginia hospital for violating the conditions of his release. But he says the system treated him like a hardened criminal. "I have been arrested on account of my disease, but I am not a felon," Denk, 44, said last week from his hospital ward. "But once you're in the system, it's less a matter of your psychiatric state than where you are in an arbitrary step system...whether you're picked up for public drunkenness or homicide."

During the administration of former governor George Allen (R), who abolished parole for felons, Virginia in 1992 created a strict system for the mentally ill who commit crimes. A team of state-appointed psychologists, social workers, police officers and security experts was formed to assess patients' safety risks and mete out an elaborate system of graduated privileges. Privileges range from going unescorted to the canteen, to working there, to a full-day pass away from the hospital. If patients are able to handle the additional responsibilities, they move up to the next level until their eventual release. Any release must ultimately be approved by a judge.

In 1994, the state clamped down on "insanity acquittees" after a Petersburg man who had pleaded insanity on murder charges escaped from Central State. Police eventually apprehended him, but because of the escape, the board became stricter on who could earn release. Before the creation of the panel, a patient's treatment team of doctors and psychologists made the decisions. Advocates have criticized the new system as too restrictive and prolonging patients' confinement even when their conditions have stabilized.

"Governor Allen had a no-nonsense attitude toward prisoners, so the mental health system developed a sensitive, reactive posture," said Evan Nelson, a clinical psychologist who served on the forensic review panel during the Allen administration. "Folks who had the misfortune to have just come into the system had their stays extended."

Doug, 44, from Chesterfield County, has spent four months in the forensic unit at Central State after pleading insanity to a charge of public indecency for putting his hands down his pants at a tanning salon. His mother, Bobby, who spoke on the condition that the family's last name not be published, said her son, who has manic depression, has been attacked twice by violent patients who broke his nose, stole his stereo headset and pounded his face. "We just had no idea he was going to be put in with hardened criminals and not be protected," his mother said, describing her son as a passive man.

Doug has been accepted at a community-based home in the Chesterfield area that will have a bed by June, his mother said, but the forensic panel has recommended that he remain at the hospital over the objections of one doctor who recommended a conditional release. Because he is an insanity acquittee, his case will not come up for another year—well after the bed becomes available. "He will just get lost in the system and never get out," Bobby said.

Morris, the director of forensic services, said violent incidents in the forensic unit are rare. He said patients can request to have their privileges increased as frequently as once a month. Morris said his agency is making changes to the forensic review program by shifting decisions on privileges and release recommendations to treatment teams in each of the state's seven psychiatric hospitals, rather than the panel based at Central State.

Sen. Janet D. Howell (D-Fairfax), a member of the crime commission, is drafting a bill she plans to introduce in the General Assembly next month that would restrict the confinement of those who plead insanity to misdemeanors to the maximum jail sentence they would have drawn had they pleaded guilty: one year. After that, a court would be required to release patients or commit them to a lower-security psychiatric hospital. The burden would be placed on the state to prove that the patient should not be released, rather than the other way around. "We sort of drifted into this situation with good intentions that didn't pan out," Howell said "It's reminiscent of 'One Flew Over the Cuckoo's Nest.' You end up in a mental institution beyond any reasonable amount of time."[14]

Lobotomy: Soul Murder as Medical Mercy

[In National Socialist Germany, psychiatrists systematically murdered mental patients, for their own good. In the United States, they murdered the souls of mental patients, for their own good. The reader must decide which doctors were more evil. Histories of lobotomy abound.[15] The following excerpt is an abbreviated, edited version of the summary in George J. Alexander's and Alan W. Scheflin's *Law and Mental Disorder.* T. S.]

"Isn't it true" [said Dr. Walter Freeman, responding to objections to his methods], "that when these poor devils [chronic mental patients] stop suffering, it is through a loss of what you call psyche...what happens to the psyche if it is not 'mercy killed?'"

These words of America's first and most influential evangelist for psychosurgery are remarkably frank, perhaps because they were spoken at a conference of his psychosurgical colleagues. Dr. Freeman may not have realized that the discussion was to be published... Freeman and [neurosurgeon, James] Watts's early observations and conclusions [were]: "General dullness, lack of initiative, disorientation and apathy were common and there were also slowness, procrastination, psychomotor retardation, laziness, and lack of interest in life... Weighing the various disadvantages against the advantages, however, they came unreservedly to the conclusion that their patients were benefited rather than handicapped by the operation..."

Lobotomy remained popular for two principal reasons, in spite of its disastrous results. First, the initial generation of psychosurgeons for the most part intended just the results they produced. In their eyes the hopeless back-ward patients suffered an existence of unspeakable horrors. If a partial death of the self was the price of release, it was not too high a price. Even the total "vegetabilization" of patients was justified by the relief it brought. Two important lobotomy researchers, discussing the subject at a National Institute of Mental Health conference...put it this way:

Dr. Harry Solomon [professor of psychiatry at Harvard]: good "vegetables"...are happier.

Dr. Harry Grundfest [professor of psychiatry at Columbia]: whether vegetables or not, they are happier...

Dr. Harry Solomon: he [the post-lobotomy patient] is much easier to take care of... The administration may feel blessed.

When Professor Harry Grundfest asked whether Professor Solomon was advocating lobotomy for the convenience of hospital administrators, Professor Robert Heath of Tulane University said: "Isn't that a valid thing to take into consideration?..." One physician who had no qualms about administrative goals was Dr. Walter Freeman. "The results," he wrote, "are usually quite good, especially from the administrative point of view... Women respond better than men, Negroes better than Whites."[16]

Notes

(Complete references for books are listed in the Bibliography)

Epigraph

1.   Dostoyevski, F., *Notes from Underground* (1864). Translated by Jessie Coulson. Harmondsworth, UK: Penguin, 1972, p. 29.

Preface

1.   Madison, J., "Speech at the Constitutional Convention," June 6, 1787, in Samples, J., "James Madison's vision of liberty," *CATO Policy Report*, 23: 1 and 10-12 (March/April), 2001; p. 12.
2.   Quoted in Deutsch, A., "The History of Mental Hygiene," in Hall, J. K., et al., eds., *One Hundred Years of American Psychiatry*, pp. 325-365; p. 335.
3.   McPherson, J. M., *Battle Cry of Freedom*, p. vii.
4.   Stephens, A. H., *Augusta Daily Constitutional*, March 30, 1861, quoted in McPherson, J. M., "Southern comfort," *New York Review of Books*, April 12, 2001, pp. 28-32; p. 28.
5.   Szasz, T. S., *Insanity.*
6.   Szasz, T. S., *Pharmacracy.*

Introduction

1.   Chesterton, G. K., http://mdemarco.web.wesleyan.edu/gkc/quotes.html.
2.   Meyer, F. S., "Lincoln and the old National Review: 'Lincoln without rhetoric,'" *National Review*, August 24, 1965, pp. 5-7; p. 5. http://www.lincolnmyth.com/without_rhetoric.html
3.   "Heresy," *Encyclopaedia Britannica*, vol. 11, pp. 429-430.
4.   *Catholic Encyclopedia*, http://www.newadvent.org/cathen/06796a.htm.
5.   For an analysis of the war on drugs as a crusade against heresy, see Szasz, T. S., *Ceremonial Chemistry.*
6.   http://es.rice.edu/ES/humsoc/Galileo/Things/inquisition.html. galileo@rice.edu, Copyright ©1995 Albert Van Helden.
7.   Ibid.
8.   *Catholic Encyclopedia*, http://www.newadvent.org/cathen/08026a.htm, emphasis added.
9.   Ibid.
10.   Szasz, T. S., *Fatal Freedom.*
11.   Jamison, K. R., "Mental illness: End the stigma, treat the disease" (Letter), *New York Times*, December 17, 1999. Internet edition.
12.   Jamison, K. R., quoted in Butterfield, F., "Massachusetts gun laws concerning mentally ill are faulted," *New York Times*, January 14, 2001, p. A18.

13. Feynman, R. P., *"What Do You Care What Other People Think?"* p. 114, and *The Pleasure of Finding Things Out*, p. 187.
14. Szasz, T. S., *Pharmacracy*, Chapters 4 and 5. Members of the Pembrokeshire Hearing Voices Club in Wales appear also to espouse this view. See the Club's pamphlet, "Mental health factfile," 1999. West Wales Action for Mental Health, Brighton Chambers, 124 Main Street, Pembroke, West Wales, SA71 4HN, UK.
15. Whitehead, A. N., *Adventures of Ideas*, p. 83.
16. Editor's choice, "Perceptions of doctors and what they do," *British Medical Journal*, 323 (October 6), 2001, Internet edition.
17. Quoted in Parker, L., "Families lobby to force care: Fight polarizes mental health community," *USA Today*; February 12, 2001. Internet edition.
18. Rachlin, S., "One right too many," *Bulletin of the American Academy of Psychiatry and the Law*, 3: 99-102, 1975; p. 100.
19. Ibid., pp. 100-102.
20. Acton, J. E. E. D., *Essays in the Study and Writing of History*, vol. 3, pp. 491, 490.
21. Ibid., pp. 490-491.
22. Szasz, T. S., *Pharmacracy.*
23. Steele, Appellant v. Hamilton County Community Mental Health Board, Appellee. [Cited as *Steele v. Hamilton Cty. Community Mental Health Bd.* (2000), 90 Ohio St. 3d 176.] http://www.sconet.state.oh.us/Communications_Office/summaries/2000/1018/. Emphasis added.
24. Baker, G., quoted in Hunter, R. and Macalpine, I., eds., *Three Hundred Years of Psychiatry*, p. 410.
25. Pinel, P., quoted in ibid., p. 609.
26. Smart, C., "Alleged insanity in the Army," *JAMA*, 33: 1098-99, 1900; "JAMA 100 years ago," *JAMA*, 284: 1901 (October 18), 2000.
27. Applebaum, A., "A history of horror," *New York Review of Books*, October 18, 2001, pp. 40-43; p. 41, emphasis added.
28. In this connection, see my remarks at the end of Chapter 5.
29. Johnson, S., *Selected Writings*, p. 114.
30. Hill, R. G., *The Total Abolition of Personal Restraint in the Treatment of the Insane*, p. 55. See also Hunter, R. and Macalpine, I., eds., *Three Hundred Years of Psychiatry, 1535-1860*, pp. 886-892.
31. Szasz, T. S., *Cruel Compassion*, especially chapters 9 and 10.
32. "Slavery," *Encyclopaedia Britannica*, 11th edition, vol. 25, pp. 216-227; p. 225.
33. Treffert, D. A., "'Dying with their rights on'" (Letter), *American Journal of Psychiatry*, 130: 1041 (September), 1973.

Chapter 1. Psychiatric Slavery

1. Quoted in Byrd, M., "Lincoln's shadow," *New York Times Book Review*, December 3, 2000, p. 102.
2. Coxe, J., Sir, "Testimony before the House of Commons Select Committee on the Operation of the Lunacy Laws (1877)," quoted in Scull, A., MacKenzie, C., and Hervey, N., *Masters of Bedlam*, p. 3.
3. Szasz, T. S., *Law, Liberty, and Psychiatry*, pp. 41-45.
4. Quoted in ibid., p. 43.
5. Quoted in ibid., p. 41.
6. Gordon, E. N., "Slavery," *Encyclopaedia Britannica*, vol. 20, pp. 628-644; p. 628.
7. Paine, T., *Common Sense* (1776), in Foner, P. S., ed., *The Life and Major Writings of Thomas Paine*, p. 3, emphasis in the original.

8.   See Eibner, J., "2 goats can free a slave in Sudan," *International Herald-Tribune*, June 29, 2001, p. 11.

9.   Davis, D. B., "Slavery—white, black, Muslim, Christian," *New York Review of Books*, July 5, 2001, pp. 51-55. See also, Davis, D. B., *The Problem of Slavery in Western Culture;* Kroger, L., *Black Slaveowners;* and Whitten, D. O., *Andrew Durnford.*

10.   Gordon, E. N., "Slavery," *Encyclopedia Britannica*, vol. 20, pp. 628-644; p. 630.

11.   Davis, D. B., "Free at last: The enduring legacy of the South's Civil War victory," *New York Times*, August 26, 2001, Internet edition.

12.   Szasz, T. S., *Psychiatric Slavery.*

13.   Satel, S., "For addicts, force is the best medicine," *Wall Street Journal*, January 7, 1998, p. 6.

14.   Szasz, T. S., *Pharmacracy.*

15.   Calhoun, J. C., "Slavery a Positive Good," Speech delivered in the United States Senate, February 6, 1837. http://douglass.speech.nwu.edu/calh_a59.htm; McPherson, J. M., *Battle Cry of Freedom*, p. 56.

16.   Davis, D. B., *The Problem of Slavery in Western Culture*, p. 186. See also Davis, D. B., *The Problem of Slavery in the Age of Revolution,* and *Slavery and Human Progress.*

17.   Quoted in Bunker, H. A., "American Psychiatric Literature During the Past One Hundred Years," in Hall, J. K., et al., eds., *One Hundred Years of American Psychiatry*, pp. 195-271; p. 206, emphasis added.

18.   Quoted in Deutsch, A., "The History of Mental Hygiene," in Hall, J. K., et al., eds., *One Hundred Years of American Psychiatry*, pp. 325-365; p. 335.

19.   Quoted in Hamilton, S. W., " The History of American Mental Hospitals," in Hall, J. K., et al., eds., *One Hundred Years of American Psychiatry*, pp. 73-166; p. 115.

20.   Quoted in Deutsch, A., "The History of Mental Hygiene," in Hall, J. K., et al., eds., *One Hundred Years of American Psychiatry*, pp. 325-365; p. 343.

21.   Zilboorg, G. and Henry, G. W., *A History of Medical Psychology,* p. 409.

22.   Creager, E., "A vicious circle," *Detroit Free Press*, October 31, 2000, pp. 8F-10F.

23.   Ibid.

24.   Ibid.

25.   Haggard, P., "Control of human action," http://www.psychol.ucl.ac.uk/patrick.haggard/c567/c5678.html.

26.   Noonan, J. T., Jr., *Persons and Masks of the Law*, p. 11.

27.   Ibid.

28.   See Weinberger, D. R., "A brain too young for good judgment," *New York Times*, March 10, 2001. Internet edition.

29.   Noonan, J. T., Jr., *Persons and Masks of the Law*, pp. 58, 20.

30.   Constitution of the United States, Article I, Section 2, Clause 3: Representatives and direct Taxes shall be apportioned among the several States which may be included within this Union, according to their respective Numbers, which shall be determined by adding to the whole Number of free Persons, including those bound to Service for a Term of Years, and...Three Fifths of all other Persons.

31.   *Robinson v. California*, 370 U. S. 660, 1962; pp. 666, 674.

32.   Noonan, J. T., Jr., *Persons and Masks of the Law*, p. 41.

33.   Quoted in ibid., p. 48.

34.   Ibid., p. 54.

35.   For example, see Moore, M. S., "Some myths about 'mental illness,'" *Archives of General Psychiatry*, 32: 1483-1497 (December), 1975.

36.   Zonana, H., "Mandated outpatient treatment: A quick fix for random violence?—Not likely," *Journal of the American Academy of Psychiatry and the Law*, 28: 124-126, 2000; p. 124.

37. Pence, G. E., *Classic Cases in Medical Ethics*, p. 364.
38. Quoted in Kraepelin, E., *One Hundred Years of Psychiatry*, p. 70. Ferdinand Autenrieth (1772-1835) had earlier written: "The doctor can never sufficiently impress upon himself and others the fact that the insane are identical in most respects to stubborn, ill-mannered children, and require stern (not cruel) treatment." Quoted in Kraepelin, E., *One Hundred Years of Psychiatry*, p. 70. See also Szasz, T. S., *The Myth of Psychotherapy*, pp. 74-76.
39. Quoted in ibid., pp. 69-70.
40. Mulligan, K., "Appeals Court upholds judge's order to medicate Capitol Hill shooter," *Psychiatric New*, 36: 2 (September 7), 2001.
41. Quoted in Hausman, K., "Judge orders medication for shooting suspect," *Psychiatric News*, 36: 18 & 43 (April 6), 2001.
42. Quoted in Szasz, T. S., *Law, Liberty, and Psychiatry*, p. 42.
43. Kupersanin, E., "Committing a loved one can be the best medicine," *Psychiatric News*, 36: 13 (September 7), 2001.
44. Mechanic, D., "Explanations of mental illness" (Editorial), *Journal of Nervous and Mental Disease*, 166: 381-386 (June), 1978; p. 381.
45. Ibid., p. 383.
46. Ibid., pp. 383, 385, emphasis added.
47. See Tarkan, L., "Debating patients' capacity to decide," *New York Times*, October 2, 2001, Internet edition.
48. Mechanic, D., "Explanations of mental illness" (Editorial), *Journal of Nervous and Mental Disease*, 166: 381-386 (June), 1978; pp. 381, 382.
49. Matthew 22: 21.
50. Pickin, M., Sampson, F., Munro, J., and Nicholl, J., "General practitioners' reasons for removing patients from their lists: Postal survey in England and Wales," *British Medical Journal*, 322: 1158-1159 (May 12), 2001; "Violence is main reason why GPs remove patients from their lists." http://bmj.com/cgi/content/full/322/7295/0/f
51. "Johns Hopkins AIDS service, TB & HIV," Hopkins-id.edu/tb_hiv/tbhiv_23.html; "Infection control," The National Center for HIV, STD, and TB Prevention, ww.cdc.gov/nchstp/od/nchstp.html; Centers for Disease Control & Prevention National Center for HIV, STD, and TB Prevention Divisions of HIV/AIDS Prevention, www.cdc.gov/hiv/pubs/facts.htm; "HIV/AIDS Introduction," www.cdcnpin.org/hiv/start.htm; "Disease control, case reporting, partner notification, counseling, testing, referral and education," www.co.pima.az.us/health/disease.htm. For further discussion, see Chapter 3.
52. Szasz, T. S., *Insanity* and *Cruel Compassion*.
53. Szasz, T. S., *Pharmacracy*.

Chapter 2. The Psychiatric Slave Status

1. Wilde, Oscar, "The soul of man under socialism," *Fortnightly Review*, February 1891, pp. 292-319. http://www.geocities.com/CapitolHill/Lobby/398/oscar.html
2. Chesterton, G. K., "What I Saw in America" (1928), quoted in http://www.the700club.org/bibleresources/theology/chesterton.
3. See Hoeller, K., "Thomas Szasz's history and philosophy of psychiatry," *Review of Existential Psychology & Psychiatry*, 23: 6-69, 1997.
4. Finkelman, P., *Slavery and the Founders*.
5. See http://library.wustl.edu/vlib/dredscott/chronology.html.
6. Taney, R. B., "Majority opinion, "Dred Scott, Plaintiff in Error, v. John F. A. Sanford, *Scott v. Sanford*, 60 U.S. 393 (1856). http://www.tourolaw.edu/patch/Scott. Subsequent quotes from Taney are from this source.

7.   Article I, Section 2.

8.   Taney, R. B., "Majority opinion," Dred Scott, Plaintiff in Error, v. John F. A. Sanford, *Scott v. Sanford*, 60 U.S. 393 (1856).

9.   http://lincoln.lib.niu.edu/498R/ronald/disso5.html

10. Dred Scott, Plaintiff in Error, v. John F. A. Sanford, "Mr. Justice Curtis dissenting," *Scott v. Sanford*, 60 U.S. 393 (1856). http://www.tourolaw.edu/patch/Scott/Curtis.html

11. http://lincoln.lib.niu.edu/498R/ronald/disso5.html

12. http://lincoln.lib.niu.edu/498R/ronald/disso5.html, emphasis added. And Dred Scott, Plaintiff in Error, v. John F. A. Sanford, "Mr. Justice McLean dissenting," *Scott v. Sanford*, 60 U.S. 393 (1856).

13. Ibid.

14. Szasz, T. S., *Law, Liberty, and Psychiatry*, Chapters 10 and 11.

15. Virtually every modern text on law and psychiatry presents and analyzes this case. See, for example, Stone, A. A., *Law, Psychiatry, and Morality,* chapter 7, and Appelbaum, P. S., *Almost a Revolution,* chapter 3. See also Gostin, L. O., *Public Health Law,* pp. 137-138. For the decision, see *Tarasoff v. Regents of the University of California*, 529 P.2d 553 (Cal. 1974); *People v. Poddar,* 518 P.2d 342 (Cal. 1974); and *Tarasoff v. Regents of the University of California,* 551 P.2d 334 (Cal. 1976).

16. Belli, M. M., "Warning of the dangerous patient: A practical approach," *American Journal of Forensic Psychiatry*, 2: 6-7, 1981-82; Szasz, T. S., "Szasz on the dangerous patient," ibid., pp. 6-7 & 17.

17. Belli, M. M., "Warning of the dangerous patient: A practical approach," *American Journal of Forensic Psychiatry*, 2: 6-7, 1981-82; p. 6.

18. Szasz, T. S., "Szasz on the dangerous patient," *American Journal of Forensic Psychiatry,* 2: 6-7 & 17, 1981-82; pp. 6-7.

19. Ibid., pp. 7 & 17; see also Szasz, T. S., *The Ethics of Psychoanalysis.*

20. St. Clair, L., "Insurance underwriting and psychiatry risk," *The American Psychoanalyst,* 35: 12, 2001; Hausman, K., "Medical association challenges legality of medical-privacy rule," *Psychiatric News,* 36: 2 (October 5), 2001.

21. Leinwand, D., "Secret-telling sparks some ethical conflicts," *USA Today,* July 30, 2001, Internet edition.

22. Appelbaum, P. S., *Almost a Revolution,* p. 92.

23. Ibid.

24. Ibid., p. 103.

25. Ibid., p. 100.

26. American Library Association, *Intellectual Freedom Manual,* p. 165.

27. Appelbaum, P. S., *Almost a Revolution,* p. 100.

28. Klotz, J. A., "Limiting the Psychotherapist-Patient Privilege: The Therapeutic Potential," in Wexler, D. B. and Winick, B. J., eds., *Law in a Therapeutic Key*, pp. 467-497; pp. 467-468, emphasis added. For a critical analysis of therapeutic jurisprudence, see Chapter 8.

29. Szasz, T. S., *The Myth of Mental Illness* and *The Myth of Psychotherapy.*

30. Klotz, J. A., "Limiting the Psychotherapist-Patient Privilege: The Therapeutic Potential," in Wexler, D. B. and Winick, B. J., eds., *Law in a Therapeutic Key*, pp. 467-497; p. 481.

31. Anderson, E., et al., "Coercive Uses of Mandatory Reporting in Therapeutic Relationships," in Wexler, D. B. and Winick, B. J., eds., *Law in a Therapeutic Key,* pp. 895-905; p. 897.

32. Ibid.

33. Szasz, T. S., *Fatal Freedom* and *Pharmacracy.*

34.   Szasz, T. S., *The Meaning of Mind*, Chapter 3.
35.   The False Memory Syndrome, like much else in psychiatry and mental health, is a fraud. See Szasz, T. S., *The Meaning of Mind*, p. 47-74.
36.   Quoted in Byrd, M., "Lincoln's shadow," *New York Times Book Review*, December 3, 2000, p. 102.
37.   Szasz, T. S., *Insanity* and *Cruel Compassion*.
38.   Ibid.
39.   For a typical story, see Max, D. T., "The cop and the therapist," *New York Times Magazine*, December 5, 2000, pp. 95-98.
40.   "Fugitive slave laws," http://www.worldbook.com/fun/aajourny/html/bh042.html.
41.   "Mental Health, Mental Retardation, and Substance Abuse Services," 1995, Chapter 9: Interstate Compact in Mental Health. http://janus.state.me.us/legis/statutes/34-B/title34-Bch90sec0.html. Subsequent quotes are from this source.
42.   Ibid.
43.   Szasz, T. S., "Voluntary mental hospitalization: An unacknowledged practice of medical fraud," *New England Journal of Medicine*, 287: 277-278 (August 10), 1972.
44.   *West Virginia Ex Rel. White v. Todd*, Supreme Court of Appeals of West Virginia (1996); 197 W. Va. 334; 475 S.E. 2d 426; quoted in Alexander, G. J. and Scheflin, A. W., *Law and Mental Disorder*, pp. 920-926; p. 923.
45.   Ibid., pp. 924-925.
46.   Hoffman, A., *Inventing Mark Twain*, p. 12.
47.   Szasz, T. S., "The sane slave: An historical note on the use of medical diagnosis as justificatory rhetoric," *American Journal of Psychotherapy*, 25: 228-239 (April), 1971; and *Insanity*, pp. 305-307.
48.   See Cain, W. E., "Angel of light: Interpreting John Brown," http://muse.jhu.edu/demo/rah/23.4cain.html; Katz, W. L., "John Brown at 2000: A white role model," http://www.williamlorenkatz.com/html/brown.html; and http://hilltophousehotel.atmyown.com/history.html.
49.   See Szasz, T. S., "On the theory of psychoanalytic treatment," *International Journal of Psychoanalysis*, 38: 166-182, 1957; "Psychoanalytic training: A socio-psychological analysis of its history and present status," *International Journal of Psychoanalysis,* 39: 598-613, 1958; and *The Ethics of Psychoanalysis.*
50.   Szasz, T. S., *The Myth of Psychotherapy;* St. Clair, L., "Insurance underwriting and psychiatry risk," *The American Psychoanalyst*, 35: 12, 2001.
51.   "MH groups join APA in issuing patient 'Bill of Rights,'" *Psychiatric News*, 32: 1 & 30 (March 21), 1997; p. 1, emphasis added.

Chapter 3. Psychiatric Slavery as Public Health

1.   Acton, J. E. E. D., *Essays in the Study and Writing of History,* vol. 3, pp. 516, 610.
2.   Quoted in Appelbaum, P. S., *Almost a Revolution,* p. 80.
3.   Green, T. H., quoted in Foley, H. A. and Sharfstein, S. S. *Madness and Government,* p. vii.
4.   Niemiec, D., "A cry for help, then disaster," *Free Press* (Detroit), March 14, 2001, pp. 1A & 7A.
5.   Detels, R. and Breslow, L., "Current Scope and Concerns in Public Health," in Holland, W. W., Detels, R., and Knox, G., eds. *Oxford Textbook of Public Health*, vol. 1, pp. 49-64; p. 49.
6.   Szasz, T. S., *Pharmacracy.*
7.   Koop, C. E. and Lundberg, G. D., "Violence in America: A public health emergency" (Editorial), *JAMA*, 267: 3076 (June 10), 1992.

8.   Cook, P. J., et al., "The medical costs of gunshot injuries in the United States," *JAMA*, 282: 447-454 (August 4), 1999; Ferry, L. H., Grissino, L. M., and Runfola, P. S., "Tobacco dependence curriculum in US undergraduate medical education," *JAMA*, 282: 825-828 (September 1), 1999.

9.   Benson, J., "Medical marchers ask: Should guns be part of patient profile?" *The New* York *Observer*, March 16, 2001, Internet edition.

10. Szasz, T. S., *The Myth of Mental Illness.*

11. Szasz, T. S., *Fatal Freedom.*

12. "Public psychiatry in the United States: What is it?" http://cpmcnet.columbia.edu/dept/pi/ppf/pub-psyc.html, emphasis added.

13. Kolb, L. C., *Noyes' Modern Clinical Psychiatry.*

14. Fann, W. E., "Review of *Madness on the Couch: Blaming the Victim in the Heyday of Psychoanalysis,* by Edward Dolnick," *American Journal of Psychiatry,* 158: 505-506, (March), 2001, emphasis added; see also Kaplan, H. I. and Sadock, B. J., *Kaplan and Sadock's Synopsis of Psychiatry.*

15. Detels, R. and Breslow, L., "Current Scope and Concerns in Public Health," in Holland, W. W., Detels, R., and Knox, G., eds. *Oxford Textbook of Public Health,* vol. 1, pp. 49-64; p. 54.

16. Szasz, T. S., *Insanity.*

17. Coker, R., *From Chaos to Coercion*, p. 204, emphasis added.

18. Ibid., p. 105, emphasis added.

19. Ibid., p. 33, emphasis added.

20. Neal, K., "Compulsory treatment for infectious disease" (Letter), *The Lancet*, 343: 675 (March 12), 1994, and Morton, M. and Marshall, R., "Public interest versus confidentiality in notifiable diseases" (Letter), *The Lancet*, 343: 359 (February 5), 1994, emphasis added.

21. Gasner, M. R., et al., "The use of legal action in New York City to ensure treatment of tuberculosis," *New England Journal of Medicine*, 340: 359-366 (February 4), 1999.

22. Ibid., p. 33.

23. Ibid., pp. 105, 111, 214, emphasis added.

24. Campion, E. W., "Liberty and the control of tuberculosis" (Editorial), *New England Journal of Medicine,* 340: 385-386 (February 4), 1999, emphasis added.

25. Hausman, K., "State can forcibly medicate nonviolent patients, Court rules," *Psychiatric News*, 36: 8 & 21 (January 5), 2001; p. 8, emphasis added.

26. Ibid.

27. Torrey, E. F. and Miller, J., "Can psychiatry learn from tuberculosis treatment?" *Psychiatric Services,* 50: 1389 (November), 1999; emphasis added.

28. Fisher, C., "Carrie Fisher: Perhaps one of manic-depression's best-known champions, the writer and actress shows us how she wrangles her many moods," *Psychology Today*, 34: 33-37 & 87 (December), 2001; p. 87.

29. Fox, V., "First person account: Schizophrenia, medication, and outpatient commitment," *Catalyst* (Treatment Advocacy Center), 3: 4-5 (July / August), 2001. Kay Redfield Jamison shares this view; see *An Unquiet Mind*, p. 113.

30. "Reportable Diseases," www.cdc.gov/nchs/SSBR/027para.htm; see also Minkoff, H. and Santoro, N., "Ethical considerations in the treatment of infertility in women with human immunodeficiency virus infection," *New England Journal of Medicine,* 342: 1748-1750 (June 8), 2000.

31. Szasz, T. S., *Ceremonial Chemistry.*

32. http://www.nps.gov/kala/docs/faq.htm

33. "The history of leprosy," http://www.webspawner.com/banner/index.html.

34. "Secret People," http://www.pbs.org/independentlens/1999/secret_interview.html.

35.   Teague, M., "A hard way home," *Times-Picayune* (New Orleans), February 4, 2001, E1 & E4-E5.
36.   CNN Networks, "Leprosy hospital's closure means new start for patients: Leprosy is now easily controllable with drugs." http://www.cnn.com/US/9804/ 24/last.lepers/
37.   ABCNews.com, "Last patients fight to stay at leprosy center," December 17, 2000. http://www.abcnews.go.com/sections/us/DailyNews/hansens990329a.html
38.   Szasz, T. S., *Insanity.*
39.   Bucknill, J. C., "Visiting physicians to county asylums," *The Asylum Journal*, 1: 33-36, 1854; in Hunter, I. and Macalpine, I., *Three Hundred Years of Psychiatry*, pp. 1010-1013; p. 1013.
40.   See Ross, C. A., "Errors in Logic in Biological Psychiatry," in Ross, C. A. and Pam, A., *Pseudoscience in Biological Psychiatry*, p. 85.
41.   Szasz, T. S., "Whither psychiatry?" [1966], in Szasz, T. S., *Ideology and Insanity*, pp. 243-244.
42.   Szasz, T. S., *Psychiatric Slavery.*
43.   Goodchild, S., "Playwright held in Broadmoor forced to take 'zombie' drugs," www.independent.co.uk, April 23, 2000.
44.   Gutheil, T. G., "In search of true freedom: Drug refusal, involuntary medication, and 'rotting with your rights on,'" *American Journal of Psychiatry*, 137: 327-28 (1980), p. 327.
45.   Peele, R. and Keisling, R., "Patient's right to receive adequate care explored," *Psychiatric News*, December 5, 1980, pp. 1 & 28; p. 28.
46.   Goffman, E., *Asylums*, p. 140.
47.   Miller, R., "The ethics of involuntary commitment to mental health treatment," in Bloch, S. and Chodoff, P., eds., *Psychiatric Ethics*, 2nd edition, pp. 265-289; p. 280, emphasis added.
48.   Jaffe, D. J., "How to prepare for an emergency," (2000), http://www.nami.org/ about/naminyc/coping/911.html. More than half a century ago, James Thurber parodied the commitment process in his short essay, "The unicorn in the garden," reprinted in Szasz, T. S., ed., *The Age of Madness*, pp. 278-279.
49.   For an acknowledgment of the importance of this consideration, see Porter, R., "Madness and Its Institutions," in Wear, A., ed., *Medicine in Society*, pp. 277-301; pp. 277-278.
50.   Quoted in Arehart-Treichel, J., "Lawyers and psychiatry experts: Not a marriage made in heaven," *Psychiatric News*, 35: 10 (December 1), 2000.
51.   Ciardi, J., in Dante, A., *The Inferno*, p. 41.
52.   Dante A., *The Inferno*, pp. 42-43.
53.   Sinclair, J. D., in Dante, A., *The Divine Comedy of Dante Alighieri*, pp. 54-55.
54.   Szasz, T. S., *Fatal Freedom.*

Chapter 4. Justifying Psychiatric Slavery

1.   Locke, J., *An Essay Concerning Human Understanding*, p. 198.
2.   Camus, A., "Homage to an Exile" (1955), in Camus, A., *Resistance, Rebellion, Death*, p. 101.
3.   Szasz, T. S., *Insanity* and *Cruel Compassion.*
4.   See Szasz, T. S., *Pharmacracy.*
5.   For an expose of the new "homes" for the mentally ill, see "The care takers," *Detroit News*, May 2, 1993, pp. 1A & 10A-13A.
6.   Blain, D., quoted in, Johnson, A. B., *Out of Bedlam*, p. 30, emphasis added.
7.   Quoted in Visotsky, H. M., "The great American roundup," *New England Journal of Medicine*, 317: 1662-1663 (December 24), 1987, p. 1963.

8. Szasz, T. S., *Psychiatric Justice.*

9. Szasz, T. S., *The Therapeutic State* and *Pharmacracy.*

10. Miller, R., "The ethics of involuntary commitment to mental health treatment," in Bloch, S. and Chodoff, P., eds., *Psychiatric Ethics,* 2nd edition, pp. 265-289.

11. Jackman, T., "Illegal home entries put police unit tactics on trial," *Washington Post,* June 26, 2000, Internet edition.

12. Quoted in Dewey, R., "The jury law for commitment of the insane in Illinois (1867-1893), and Mrs. E. P. W. Packard, its author, also later developments in lunacy legislation in Illinois," *American Journal of Insanity,* 69: 571-584 (January), 1913; for details, see Szasz, T. S., *The Manufacture of Madness,* pp. 15, 130-132.

13. *Kansas v. Leroy Hendricks, No. 95-1649.* "Excerpts from opinions on status of sex offenders," *New York Times,* June 24, 1997, p. B11.

14. Associated Press, "Jury: 95-year-old sexual predator is still a threat," *Syracuse Herald-Journal,* February 2, 2000, p. A8.

15. Stone, A. A., *Law, Psychiatry, and Morality,* p. 140.

16. La Fond, J. Q. and Durham, M. L., *Back to the Asylum,* pp. 170-171.

17. Sandford, J. J., "Public health psychiatry and crime prevention," *British Medical Journal,* May 15, 1999. http://www.findarticles.com/m0999/7194_318/54851600/p1/article.jhtml

18. Editorial, *British Medical Journal,* May 15, 1999. http://www.findarticles.com/m0999/7194_318/54851600/p1/article.jhtml ibid., emphasis added.

19. Szmukler, G. and Holloway, F., "Mental health legislation is now a harmful anachronism," *Psychiatric Bulletin,* 22: 662-665, 1998. For a similar proposal, see Fishman, R., "Israeli psychiatrists propose new law for forced incarceration of patients," *The Lancet,* 357: 1956 (June 16), 2001. Internet edition.

20. Szmukler, G. and Holloway, F., "Mental health legislation is now a harmful anachronism," *Psychiatric Bulletin,* 22: 662-665, 1998.

21. Quoted in Sayce, L., "Transcending mental health law," *Psychiatric Bulletin,* 22: 669-670, 1998.

22. Szasz, T. S., *The Myth of Mental Illness*; see also Szasz, T. S., "Mental illness: Psychiatry's phlogiston," *Journal of Medical Ethics,* 27: 297-301, 2001.

23. Szasz, T. S., *Cruel Compassion,* Chapter 3.

24. Grasset, J. *The Semi-Insane and the Semi-Responsible,* pp. 368-369, emphasis added.

25. Menninger, K., *The Crime of Punishment,* pp. 257, 260.

26. Quoted in Ramsay, S., "UK psychiatrists refuse to treat the untreatable," *The Lancet,* 353: 647 (February 20), 1999.

27. "Mentally ill detention plans backed," BBC World Service, 14 March, 2000, Internet edition.

28. "New police unit will target would-be killers," *Sunday Times* (London), July 1, 2001, p. 1/3.

29. Quoted in Ramsay, S., "UK psychiatrists refuse to treat the untreatable," *The Lancet,* 353: 647 (February 20), 1999, emphasis added.

30. Ibid., emphasis added.

31. Eastman, N., "Public health psychiatry or crime prevention?" (Editorial), *British Medical Journal,* 318: 549-550 (February 27), 1999; p. 550, emphasis added.

32. Pinard, G.F. and Pagani, L., eds., *Clinical Assessment of Dangerousness.*

33. Feynman, R. P., *The Pleasure of Findings Things Out.*

34. Szasz, T. S., *Insanity.*

35. Simon, R. I., "Review of *Clinical Assessment of Dangerousness,*" *JAMA,* vol. 286, October 10, 2001; http://jama.ama-assn.org/issues/current/ffull/jbk1010-2.html.

36. Palmstierna, T., "Only about 1 in 30 predictions of assault by discharged psychiatric patients will be correct," *British Medical Journal*, 319: 1270 (November 6), 1999.

37. Maden, A., "Book review," *Psychiatric Bulletin*, 24: 37-39, 2000. Subsequent references are to this source.

38. Quoted in Morris, T. D., *Southern Slavery and the Law*, p. 229.

39. Szasz, T., S., *Fatal Freedom*, especially pp. 45-62; Davies, S., "Assaults and threats on psychiatrists," *Psychiatric Bulletin*, 25: 89-91, 2001; p. 89.

40. Quoted from the *Journal of Mental Science*, volume 110, January 1898, in "One hundred years ago," *British Journal of Psychiatry*, 74: 79 (April) 1999.

Chapter 5. Jim Crow Psychiatry I

1. Maine, H. S., *Ancient Law*, pp. 163-165, emphasis in the original.

2. Oakeshott, M., quoted in Hartwell, R. M., "Introduction," in Templeton, K. S., Jr., ed., *The Politicization of Society*, p. 20.

3. http://www.usbol.com/ctjournal/JCrow1.html and http://www.toptags.com/aama/docs/jcrow.htm

4. O'Brien, M., "Jim Crow was there," *TLS* (London), May 25, 2001, pp. 13-14.

5. Appelbaum, P. S., *Almost a Revolution*, p. 119, emphasis added.

6. Gutheil, T. G., "In search of true freedom: Drug refusal, involuntary medication, and 'rotting with your rights on'" (Editorial), *American Journal of Psychiatry*, 137: 327-328 (April), 1980; p. 328, emphasis added.

7. Peele, R. and Keisling, R., "Patient's right to receive adequate care explored,"*Psychiatric News*, December 5, 1980, pp. 1 & 28; p. 28, emphasis added.

8. "Patient's right to receive adequate care explored," *Psychiatric News*, December 5, 1980, pp. 1 & 28; p. 1, emphasis added.

9. Jaspers, K., *General Psychopathology*, pp. 839-840.

10. See "Minnesota Advance Psychiatric Directive and Health Care Directive," http://www.mnlegalservices.org/publications/MDLC20Fact20Sheets/apd_healthdirective.html.

11. Szasz, T. S., "The psychiatric will: A new mechanism for protecting persons against 'psychosis' and psychiatry," *American Psychologist*, 37: 762-770 (July), 1982; "The psychiatric will: II. Whose will is it anyway?" *American Psychologist*, 38: 344-346 (March), 1983; and "The Psychiatric Will," in Szasz, T. S., *A Lexicon of Lunacy*, pp. 159-172.

12. Alexander, G. J. and Szasz, T. S., "From contract to status via psychiatry," *Santa Clara Lawyer*, 13: 537-559 (Spring), 1973.

13. Tuttle, J., "Voter restriction unconstitutional: Ruling lets mentally ill cast ballots," *Bangor Daily News* (Maine), August 11, 2001, p. 1.

14. See, for example, Appelbaum, P. S., *Almost a Revolution*; Bloch, S. and Chodoff, P., eds, *Psychiatric Ethics*; Stone, A. A., *Law, Psychiatry and Morality;* and Szasz, T. S., *Insanity.*

15. Chodoff, P. and Peele, R., "A wary view of a new testament: The psychiatric will of Dr. Szasz," *Hastings Center Report*, 13: 11-13 (April) 1983; pp. 13, 12.

16. Keisling, R., "Turning back the clock: A response to Szasz," ibid., p. 343.

17. See Szasz, T. S., *Law, Liberty, and Psychiatry* and *Psychiatric Justice*; see also Appendix II in this volume.

18. Winick, B. J., "Advance directive instruments for those with mental illness," *University of Miami Law Review,* 51: 57-95, 1996; p. 95, emphasis added.

19. Ibid., p. 68, emphasis added.

20. Ibid., p. 73.

21. Winick, B. J., *The Right to Refuse Mental Health Treatment* , pp. 398-399.

22. See Chapter 3.
23. See Winick, B. J., "Advance directive instruments for those with mental illness," *University of Miami Law Review,* 51: 57-95, 1996; p. 81.
24. Miller, R. D., "Advance directives for psychiatric treatment: A view from the trenches," *Psychology, Public Policy, and Law,* 4: 728-745, 1998; p. 745, emphasis added.
25. Halpern, A. and Szmukler, G., " Psychiatric advance directives: Reconciling autonomy and non-consensual treatment," *Psychiatric Bulletin,* 21: 323-327, 1997; p. 323, emphasis added.
26. Ibid., p. 326, emphasis added.
27. Quoted in Butterfield, F., "Massachusetts gun laws concerning mentally ill are faulted," *New York Times,* January 14, 2001, Internet edition. Regarding this issue, see Szasz, T. S., "An 'Unscrewtape' letter: A reply to Fred Sander," *American Journal of Psychiatry,* 125: 1432-1435 (April), 1969. See also "Community discussion: Should volunteering be mandatory?" *Los Angeles Times,* March 31, 2001, p. B9.
28. Jamison, K. R., *An Unquiet Mind,* p. 113.
29. Widdershoven, G. and Berghmans, R., "Advance directives in psychiatric care: A narrative approach," *Journal of Medical Ethics,* 27: 92-07, 2001.
30. Ibid.
31. Savulescu, J. and Dickenson, D., "The time frame of preferences, dispositions, and the validity of advance directives for the mentally ill," *Philosophy, Psychiatry & Psychology,* 5: 225-246 (September) 1998; p. 225.
32. Ibid., pp. 239, 241, emphasis added.
33. Associated Press, "Gunman shoots 2 deputies, 1 fatally, then kills himself," *Syracuse Herald-Journal,* April 28, 2001, p. A2. See also Szasz, T. S., *Fatal Freedom,* chapter 4.
34. Quoted in Turner, E. S., "The accoucheur's son," *Times Literary Supplement,* March 23, 2001, p. 36.
35. Fredrickson, G. M., "The skeleton in the closet," *New York Review of Books,* November 2, 2000, pp. 61-65; p. 63.
36. Jefferson, T., "Letter to Edward Coles, August 25, 1814," quoted in Finkelman, P., *Slavery and the Founders,* p. 196.
37. Marks, J., *The Search for the "Manchurian Candidate."*
38. See McIlroy, A., "When depression turns deadly: Can antidepressants transform despair into suicide?" *The Globe and Mail* (Toronto), April 21, 2001, Internet edition; Atwater, A., "Correlation seen between antidepressants, violence," September 10, 2001, mhttp://www.news-press.com/news/today/010909antidepressant.html; Rosack, J., "SSRIs called on carpet over violence claims," *Psychiatric News,* 36: 8 & 31 (October 5), 2001; "The David Healy affair," http://www.pharmapolitics.com/

Chapter 6. Jim Crow Psychiatry II

1. Macauley, T. B., quoted in Coker, R., *From Chaos to Coercion,* p. 83. Baron (Thomas Babington) Macauley (1800-1859)—English historian, essayist, and statesman—fought for the abolition of slavery as an ally of William Wilberforce, the leading English abolitionist.
2. Chekhov, A., "Ward No., 6," in *Seven Short Stories by Chekhov,* p. 130.
3. Kennedy, J. F., "Message from the President of the United States relative to mental illness and mental retardation." February 5, 1963. 88th Congress, 1st session. H. Rep. Document No. 58.
4. Quoted in Office of the Press Secretary of the President of the United States, "Remarks by the President, the First Lady, the Vice President, and Mrs. Gore at

White House Conference on Mental Health," Blackburn Auditorium, Howard University, Washington. D.C., June 7, 1999. Arianna Online, 1158 26th Street, Suite #428, Santa Monica, CA 90403, E-mail: info@ariannaonline.com, Copyright © 1998 Christabella, Inc.

5.   Clinton, H. R., ibid.
6.   Ibid., emphasis added.
7.   "Campaign moves Congress and the nation forward," *Campaign Spotlight* (The Quarterly NAMI Review), vol. 1, No. 2, 1997.
8.   Szasz, T. S., *The Meaning of Mind.*
9.   http://www.nami.org. Copyright © 1996-98 NAMI—All Rights Reserved, April 1998.
10.   "Campaign moves Congress and the nation forward," *Campaign Spotlight* (The Quarterly NAMI Review), vol. 1, No. 2, 1997.
11.   Thomson, W. T., et al., "Challenge of culture, conscience, and contract to general practitioners' care of their own health: Qualitative study," *British Medical Journal*, 323: 728-731 (September 29), 2001; http://bmj.com/cgi/content/full/323/7315/728.
12.   Editorial, "Equitable coverage for mental illness," *New York Times*, June 10, 1999, p. A30.
13.   Editorial, "The Patient Self-Determination Act," *JAMA*, 266: 410-412 (July 17), 1991.
14.   Greco, P. J. et al., "The patient self-determination act and the future of advance directives," *Annals of Internal Medicine*, 115: 639-643 (October 15), 1991; emphasis added.
15.   This volume, Introduction and Chapter 5; and see Jamison, K. R., *An Unquiet Mind*, pp. 112-113.
16.   Parker, L., "'Psychotic,' but is Andrea Yates legally insane?" *USA Today*, September 11, 2001. http://www.usatoday.com/hphoto.htm#more
17.   Ulrich, L. P., *The Patient Self-Determination Act*, p. 10, emphasis added.
18.   See Chapter 4.
19.   Ulrich, L. P., *The Patient Self-Determination Act*, p. 12.
20.   Szasz, T. S., *Insanity.*
21.   Cited in Appelbaum, P. S., *Almost a Revolution*, p. 117.
22.   *Union Pacific Railway Co. v. Botsford,* 141 U.S. 250, 251, 1891.
23.   Brandeis, L., *Olmstead v. United States*, 277 U.S. 438, 1928; p. 479.
24.   Burger, W., *Application of President and Directors of Georgetown College*, 331 F. 2nd, 1010, D.C. Cir., 1964; emphasis in the original.
25.   Callahan, L. A. and Silver, E., "Factors associated with the conditional release of persons acquitted by reason of insanity," *Law and Human Behavior*, 22: 147-163, 1998; p. 149.
26.   Thoreau, H. D., "Slavery in Massachusetts," address delivered at an Anti-Slavery Celebration, at Framingham, Massachusetts, on July 4, 1854, after the conviction in Boston of fugitive slave Anthony Burns. http://eserver.org/thoreau/slavery.html
27.   "Emancipation Proclamation," http://www.nara.gov/exhall/featured-document/eman/emanproc.html.
28.   Winick, B. J., "Advance directive instruments for those with mental illness," *University of Miami Law Review,* 51: 57-95, 1996. http://www.brucewinick.com/Abstract_ADI_for_Mental_Illness.htm
29.   Ibid.
30.   The following articles were all published before 1970. Szasz, T. S., "Commitment of the mentally ill: 'Treatment' or social restraint? *Journal of Nervous and Mental Disease,* 125: 293-307 (Apr.-June), 1957; "Psychiatry, ethics, and the criminal law," *Columbia Law Review,* 58: 183-198 (Feb.), 1958; "Moral conflict and psy-

chiatry," *Yale Review*, 49: 555-566 (June), 1960; "Open doors or civil rights for mental patients?" *Journal of Individual Psychology*, 18: 168-171 (Nov.), 1962; *Law, Liberty, and Psychiatry;* "Criminal insanity: Fact or strategy?" *New Republic*, November 21, 1964, pp. 19-22; *Psychiatric Justice;* "Toward the therapeutic state," *New Republic,* December 11, 1965, pp. 26-29; "Problems Facing Psychiatry: The Psychiatrist as Party to Conflict," in Torrey, E. F., ed., *Ethical Issues in Medicine*, pp. 265-284; "Review of *The Insanity Defense,* by Abraham S. Goldstein, and *Criminal Justice*, by Abraham S. Blumberg," *Boston University Law Review,* 48: 151-155 (Winter), 1968; "Justice and psychiatry," *Atlantic,* October, 1968, pp. 127-132; "Mental illness as an excuse for civil wrongs," (with George J. Alexander), *Journal of Nervous and Mental Disease,* 147: 113-123 (Aug.), 1968; "Science and public policy: The crime of involuntary mental hospitalization," *Medical Opinion & Review,* 4: 24-35 (May), 1968; "Subversion of the rule of law," *National Review*, March 12, 1968, pp. 247-248; "The crime of commitment," *Psychology Today*, 2: 55-57 (March), 1969.

31.   Winick, *B. J., The Right to Refuse Mental Health Treatment.*

32.   Gallagher, E. M., "Advance directives for psychiatric case: A theoretical and practical overview for legal professionals," *Psychology, Public Policy, and Law,* 4: 746-787, 1998; p. 758.

33.   Ibid., p. 775, emphasis added.

34.   "Health-care proxy," *The Columbia Encyclopedia*, Sixth Edition, 2000. http://www.bartleby.com/65/he/health-ca.html, emphasis added.

35.   Office of the New York State Attorney General, "Health care proxy." http://www.oag.state.ny.us/health/care_proxy.html. http://www.health.state.ny.us/nysdoh/hospital/proxy.htm. Emphasis added.

36.   Partnership for Caring, "Advance directives: Living wills, durable power of attorney for health care." http://www.choices.org/ad.htm

37.   The Minnesota Disability Law Center, "Minnesota advance psychiatric directive and health care directive." http://www.mnlegalservices.org/publications/MDLC20Fact20Sheets/apd_healthdirective.html. © 2000 Minnesota Legal Services Coalition.

38.   Quoted from *Quarterly Review* (London), April 1901, in Darnton, R., "Extraordinary commonplaces," *New York Review of Books*, December 21, 2000, pp.82-87; p. 82.

39.   Vogel-Scibilia, S., "Preparing an advance directive." http://namipa.nami.org/about/amipa/winter99/AdvanceDir.html

40.   Kasper, J. A., et al., "Prospective study of patients' refusal of antipsychotic medication under a physician discretion review procedure," *American Journal of Psychiatry*, 154: 483-489 (April), 1997.

41.   Hugo, V., quoted in *Bartlett's Familiar Quotations*, 16th ed., p. 427.

42.   Byrne, P., "Psychiatric stigma," *British Journal of Psychiatry*, 178: 281-284, 2001; Crisp, A., "The tendency to stigmatize," ibid., pp. 197-199.

43.   See for example, Blackmon, D. A., "After U.S. Civil War, slavery endured under a new name: 'Convict-leasing' lasted well into the 20th century," *Wall Street Journal Europe*, July 16, 2001, pp. 1 & 8.

44.   Amering, M., et al., "Psychiatric wills of mental health professionals: A survey of opinions regarding advance directives in psychiatry," *Social Psychiatry and Epidemiology,* 34: 30-34, 1999.

45.   Acton, J. E. E. D., "Letter to Johann Joseph Ignaz Dollinger, June 16, 1882," in Acton, J. E. E. D., *Essays in the Study and Writing of History*, vol. 3, pp. 665-674; pp. 667, 669, 670.

Chapter 7. Expanding Psychiatric Slavery

1. Fitzhugh, G., "The blessings of slavery," http://longman.awl.com/garraty/primarysource_10_5.htm.
2. Acton, J. E. E. D., *Essays in the Study and Writing of History*, Vol. 3, p. 516.
3. Sharfstein, S. S., "The case for caring coercion," *The New Psychiatric Review* (Sheppard Pratt Health System), 3: 1-4 (April), 2001. "The coercion must be a caring one insofar as there is present a panoply of services—a full hospital without walls."
4. Carlson, P., "Thinking outside the box: E. Fuller Torrey has brains," *Washington Post,* April 9, 2001, p. C1. http://www.washingtonpost.com/wp-dyn/articles/A57664-2001Apr8.html
5. Gerbasi, J. B., Bonnie, R. J., and Binder, R. L., "Resource document on mandatory outpatient treatment," *Journal of the American Academy of Psychiatry and Law,* 28: 127-144, 2000; p. 127.
6. Ibid. , emphasis added.
7. Gerbasi, J. B., Bonnie, R. J., and Binder, R. L., "Resource document on mandatory outpatient treatment," *Journal of the American Academy of Psychiatry and Law,* 28: 127-144, 2000; p. 129.
8. Torrey, E. F. and Kaplan, R. J., "A national survey of outpatient commitment," *Psychiatric Services,* 46: 778-784 (August), 1995. See also Parker, L., "Families lobby to force care: Fight polarizes mental health community," *USA Today;* February 12, 2001, Internet edition; and Zonana, H., "Mandated outpatient treatment: A quick fix for random violence?—Not likely," *Journal of the American Academy of Psychiatry and Law,* 28: 124-128, 2000; p. 125.
9. Benford, T. L., "Outpatient civil commitment in New York: An update," *Bulletin of the New York State Psychiatric Association,* 44: 6 (Sprig), 2001.
10. Ibid., p. 126.
11. Szasz, T. S., *Heresies,* p. 161. See also Szasz, T. S., *Schizophrenia.*
12. Korman, H., Engster, D., and Milstein, B. M., "Housing as a Tool of Coercion," in Dennis, D. L. and Monahan, J., *Coercion and Aggressive Community Treatment,* pp. 95-113.
13. Borum, R., et al., "Consumer perceptions of involuntary outpatient commitment," *Psychiatric Services,* 50: 1489-1491 (November), 1999, p. 1490, emphasis added.
14. See Gomory, T., "Coercion justified?—Evaluating the training in community living model: A conceptual and empirical critique," Ph.D. Dissertation, 1998. http://home.att.net/~PatRisser/force/PACTdissertation.html
15. Ridgely, M. S., Borum, R., and Petrila, J., *The Effectiveness of Involuntary Outpatient Treatment,* and Rand Corporation, "Does involuntary outpatient treatment work?" *Rand Law & Health Research Brief* (RB-4537), 2001, pp. 1-4.
16. Ridgely, M. S., Borum, R., and Petrila, J., *The Effectiveness of Involuntary Outpatient Treatment,* p. ix.
17. See Goffman, E., *Asylums.*
18. Ridgely, M. S., Borum, R., and Petrila, J., *The Effectiveness of Involuntary Outpatient Treatment,* p. x, emphasis added.
19. Ibid.
20. Ibid., p. ix.
21. Quoted in Parker, L., "Families lobby to force care: Fight polarizes mental health community," *USA Today;* February 12, 2001. Internet edition.
22. Carlson, P., "Thinking outside the box: E. Fuller Torrey has brains," *Washington Post,* April 9, 2001, p. C1. http://www.washingtonpost.com/wp-dyn/articles/A57664-2001Apr8.html

23. Satel, S., "Real help for the mentally ill," *New York Times*, January 7, 1999. Internet edition. Http://www.eppc.org/publications/xq/ASP/pubsID.63/qx/pubs_viewdetail.htm, emphasis added.
24. Hoyer, G., "On the justification for civil commitment," *Acta Psychiatrica Scandinavica*, 101: 65-71, 2000, pp. 70, 65.
25. *Donaldson v. O'Connor*, 493 F 2d, 507, 1974, p. 518; see Szasz, T. S., *Psychiatric Slavery*, p. 30.
26. *Donaldson v. O'Connor*, 493 F 2d, 507, 1974, p. 510; see Szasz, T. S., *Psychiatric Slavery*, p. 31.
27. Torrey, E. F., et al., *Criminalizing the Seriously Mentally Ill.*
28. U. S. Public Health Service, *Report of the Surgeon General's Conference on Children's Mental Health: A National Action Agenda.* Washington, D.C., 2000, p. 13. Satcher is a mouthpiece for the APA and the drug industry. See Satcher, D., "Special Advertising Feature: Mental Health—Sound Advice For Everyone: Mental Illnesses—Real Diseases, Real Treatments," Time, June 4, 2001, 10 pages advertising psychotropic prescription drugs.
29. Jackson, J., "What *ought* psychology to do?" *American Psychologist*, 55: 328-330 (March), 2000; p. 300.
30. Kupersanin, E., "Outpatient commitment law becomes N.Y. battleground," *Psychiatric News*, 35: 7 & 33 (August 18), 2000.
31. See Healy, D., *The Antidepressant Era*; Ross, C. and Pam, A., *Pseudoscience in Biological Psychiatry*; Bassman, R., "Whose reality is it anyway? Consumers/survivors/ex-patients speak for themselves," *Journal of Humanistic Psychology*, 41: 11-35 (Fall), 2001; and Breggin, P. R., "Empathic self-transformation and love in individual and family therapy," *The Humanistic Psychologist*, 27: 267-282 (Autumn), 1999.
32. Chesler, P., "Foreword," in Geller, J, L. and Harris, M., eds., *Women of the Asylum*, pp. xiii-xxvii; pp. xxiv-xxv.
33. NAMI E-News, September 22, 2000, Vol. 01-20. http://www.nami.org/update/enewslist.htm, emphasis added.
34. Ibid.
35. Sharfstein, S. S., "The case for caring coercion," *The New Psychiatric Review* (Sheppard Pratt Health System), 3: 1-4 (April), 2001; p. 1.
36. Ibid., emphasis added.
37. Lion, J. R., "Please make the mental patient go away," *The New Psychiatric Review* (Sheppard Pratt Health System), 3: 3 (April), 2001.
38. In this connection, see the British magazine *Asylums: The Magazine for Democratic Psychiatry* and http://asylum-online.net.
39. See Szasz, T. S., *Cruel Compassion* and the references therein.
40. Monahan, J., "From the man who brought you deinstitutionalization," *Contemporary Psychology*, 33: 492 (June), 1988; see also Isaac, R. J. and Armat, V. C., *Madness in the Streets.*
41. Szasz, T. S., *Law, Liberty, and Psychiatry.*
42. Monahan, J., "From the man who brought you deinstitutionalization," *Contemporary Psychology*, 33: 492 (June), 1988.
43. Bublis, M. D., "Szasz award" (Letters), *Psychiatric News*, 25: 16 (May 15), 1992.
44. Isaac, R. J. and Armat, V. C., *Madness in the Streets*, pp. 14-15; Isaac, R. J. and Armat, V. C., "'Right' to madness: A cruel hoax," *Los Angeles Times*, December 5, 1990.
45. Isaac, R. J. and Armat, V. C., *Madness in the Streets*, p. 155.
46. Gutheil, T. G., "Letter to Dr. Jeffrey Schaler," April 18, 2001; www.szasz.com.
47. Sharfstein, S. S., "The impact of the mentally ill offender on the criminal justice

system," Testimony for the US House Subcommittee on Crime, House Judiciary Committee, September 21, 2000. http://www.house.gov/judiciary/shar0921.htm, emphasis added.

48. Ibid.
49. Ibid., and Sharfstein, S. S., quoted in http://www.psychlaws.org/.
50. Szasz, T. S., "State mental hospitals: Orphanages for adults," *Pacific News Service Syndicate*, February 23, 1978.
51. Szasz, T. S., *Cruel Compassion*, especially chapters 9 and 10.
52. *Le Forum* (Arles), December 30, 1888; quoted in *Genius Ignored*, Chapter 7: Van Gogh, http://www.serve.com/Lucius/VanGogh.index.html.
53. Van Gogh, V., *Dear Theo,* p. 416.
54. Ibid.
55. Ibid., p. 417.
56. Ibid., pp. 422, 425, 428.
57. Quoted in quoted in *Genius Ignored*, Chapter 7: Van Gogh, http://www.serve.com/Lucius/VanGogh.index.html.
58. Van Gogh, V., *Dear Theo,* pp. 186, 256, 381. Emphasis added.
59. Quoted in *Genius Ignored*, Chapter 7: Van Gogh, http://www.serve.com/Lucius/VanGogh.index.html. Subsequent quotes are from this source, unless otherwise indicated.
60. Winchester, S., *The Professor and the Madman*, p. 44.
61. Ibid., p. 49.
62. Ibid., p. 70.
63. Ibid., p. 12.
64. Ibid., pp. 20, 21.
65. Ibid., p. 120.
66. Winchester, S., "The First Meeting between James Murray and William Chester Minor: Some New Evidence," http://www.oed.com/public/news/9806.htm#WCMinor.
67. Quoted in Winchester, S., *The Professor and the Madman*, p. 176.
68. Ibid., p. 178.
69. Coetzee, J. M., "The genius of Robert Walser," *New York Review of Books,* November 2, 2000, pp. 13-16; p. 14.
70. Quoted in ibid., p. 13.
71. Walser, R., "Letter to Therese Breitbach, 24 December 1929. www.cx.unibe.ch/hist/hifa/sites/personen/Walser.html. My translation.
72. Cavelty, G., *"Wo Bescheidenheit spaziert"* ("Where modesty strolls"), *Neue Zürcher Zeitung*, August 4, 2001, p. 17.
73. Stein, L. I. and Santos, A. B., *Assertive Community Treatment of Persons with Severe Mental Illness,* p. 102.
74. Szasz, T. S., *Pharmacracy.*
75. "Community discussion: Should volunteering be mandatory?" *Los Angeles Times*, March 31, 2001, p. B9.
76. Ibid., emphasis added.

Chapter 8. Glorifying Psychiatric Slavery

1. Kipling, R., "The white man's burden," *McClure's Magazine* , February 12, 1899; http://www.boondocksnet.com/kipling/kipling.html.
2. Camus, A., *The Rebel*, p. 4.
3. Tocqueville, A. de, quoted in, Auden, W. H. and Kronenberger, L., eds., *The Viking Book of Aphorisms*, p. 297.
4. See Morris, T. D., *Southern Slavery and the Law, 1619-1860.*

5. Friedman, M., quoted in Kane, J. L., "How effective is the current drug policy?" Speech before the University of Denver Faculty Forum, May 3, 2001. list@psychedelic-library.org. John L. Kane is United States Senior District Judge.

6. See Szasz, T. S., *The Ethics of Psychoanalysis.*

7. Szasz, T. S., "Some observations on the relationship between psychiatry and the law," *A.M.A. Archives of Neurology and Psychiatry*, 75: 297-315, (March), 1956; "Commitment of the mentally ill: 'Treatment' or social restraint?" *Journal of Nervous and Mental Disease*, 125: 293-307 (April-June), 1957; "Psychiatric expert testimony: Its covert meaning and social function," *Psychiatry*, 20: 313-316 (August), 1957; "The concept of testamentary capacity: Further observations on the role of psychiatric concepts in legal situations," *Journal of Nervous and Mental Disease*, 125: 474-477 (July-September), 1957; "Review of *The Criminal, the Judge, and the Public*, by Franz Alexander and Hugo Staub," *A.M.A. Archives of Neurology and Psychiatry*, 78: 109-111, (July), 1957; "Psychiatry, ethics, and the criminal law," *Columbia Law Review*, 58: 183-198 (February), 1958; "Recent books on the relation of psychiatry to criminology," *Psychiatry*, 21: 307-319 (August), 1958; "Politics and mental health: Some remarks apropos of the case of Mr. Ezra Pound," *American Journal of Psychiatry*, 115: 508-511 (December), 1958; "Pound, politics and mental health" (Letters), *American Journal of Psychiatry*, 115: 1040-1041 (May), 1959.

8. See Hoeller, K., "Thomas Szasz's history and philosophy of psychiatry," *Review of Existential Psychology & Psychiatry*, 23: 6-69, 1997; and Leifer, R., "The psychiatric repression of Dr. Thomas Szasz: Its social and political significance," ibid., pp. 85-106.

9. Szasz, T. S., "Some observations on the use of tranquilizing agents," *A.M.A. Archives of Neurology and Psychiatry*, 77: 86-92 (January), 1957; p. 91.

10. Szasz, T. S., "Psychiatry, ethics, and the criminal law," *Columbia Law Review*, 58: 183-198 (February), 1958; "Hospital refusal to release mental patient," *Cleveland Marshall Law Review*, 9: 220-226 (May), 1960; "Civil liberties and the mentally ill," *Cleveland-Marshall Law Review*, 9: 399-416 (September), 1960; "The insanity plea and the insanity verdict," *Temple Law Quarterly*, 40: 271-282 (Spring-Summer), 1967; and "The right to health," *Georgetown Law Journal*, 57: 734-751 (March), 1969.

11. Goffman, E., *Asylums*, p. 156.

12. Szasz, T. S., "American Association for the Abolition of Involuntary Mental Hospitalization," (Letter), *American Journal of Psychiatry*, 127: 1698 (June), 1971; "The American Association for the Abolition of Involuntary Mental Hospitalization," *The Abolitionist*, 1: 1-2 (Summer), 1971. See also www.szasz.org; Martindale, D. and Martindale, E., *Psychiatry and the Law.*

13. Szasz, T. S., "A.A.A.I.M.H.—R.I.P.," *The Abolitionist*, 9: 1 & 4 (September) 1979; Robinson, G., "The end of the beginning," ibid., pp. 1-2.

14. Szasz, T. S., *Sex by Prescription.*

15. Ibid., pp. 52-54.

16. Krafft-Ebing, R. von, *Psychopathia Sexualis*, pp. vi, vii.

17. Ibid., p. vii.

18. Ibid., emphasis added.

19. Freud, S., *The Psychopathology of Everyday Life* (1901), in SE, Vol. VI.

20. Szasz, T. S., "Freud as a leader," *Antioch Review*, 23: 133-144 (Summer), 1963; and *Anti-Freud.*

21. Menninger, K., *The Vital Balance.*

22. Freud, S., *The Psychopathology of Everyday Life*, SE., Vol. VI, p. 254.

23. Ibid., emphasis added.

24. Szasz, T. S., *Psychiatric Justice.*
25. Szasz, T. S., *The Manufacture of Madness, Ideology and Insanity, The Untamed Tongue.*
26. Szasz, T. S., *The Manufacture of Madness* and *Pharmacracy.*
27. Wexler, D. B. and Winick, B. J., "Introduction," in Wexler, D. B. and Winick, B. J., eds., *Law in a Therapeutic Key*, pp. xvii-xx; p. xvii.
28. Winick, B. J., "The Jurisprudence of Therapeutic Jurisprudence," in Wexler, D. B. and Winick, B. J., eds., *Law in a Therapeutic Key*, pp. 645-668; p. 646.
29. Wiethoff, W. E., *A Peculiar Humanism*, p. 154.
30. Quoted in ibid., p. 56.
31. Wexler, D. B. and Winick, B. J., "Introduction," in Wexler, D. B. and Winick, B. J., eds., *Law in a Therapeutic Key*, pp. xvii-xx; p. xvii.
32. Winick, B. J., "The Jurisprudence of Therapeutic Jurisprudence," in Wexler, D. B. and Winick, B. J., eds., *Law in a Therapeutic Key*, pp. 645-668; p. 653.
33. Ibid., p. 666.
34. See especially Szasz, T. S., *Law, Liberty, and Psychiatry, Psychiatric Justice,* and *The Age of Madness.*
35. Winick, B. J., "The Jurisprudence of Therapeutic Jurisprudence," in Wexler, D. B. and Winick, B. J., eds., *Law in a Therapeutic Key*, pp. 645-668; pp. 653-654, 666, emphasis added.
36. Ibid., pp. 657, 659.
37. Wiethoff, W. E., *A Peculiar Humanism*, pp. 158, 163.
38. Rachlin, S., "One right too many," *Bulletin of the American Academy of Psychiatry and the Law*, 3: 99-102, 1975; p. 102.
39. Tardiff, K., "Introduction," in Tardiff, K., ed., *The Psychiatric Uses of Seclusion and Restraint*, pp. xi-xv; p. xiv.
40. Szasz, T. S., *Fatal Freedom.*
41. Gutheil, T. G. and Tardiff, K., "Indications and Contraindications for Seclusion and Restraint," in Tardiff, K., ed., *The Psychiatric Uses of Seclusion and Restraint*, pp. 11-17; p. 13.
42. Wexler, D. B., "Legal Aspects of Seclusion and Restraint," in Tardiff, K., ed., *The Psychiatric Uses of Seclusion and Restraint*, pp. 111-124; p. 123.
43. Quoted in Wiethoff, W. E., *A Peculiar Humanism*, p. 146.
44. Tardiff, K., "Introduction," in Tardiff, K., ed., *The Psychiatric Uses of Seclusion and Restraint*, pp. xi-xv; p. xi-xiii.
45. Ibid., p. xiii.
46. Soloff, P. H., "Historical Notes on Seclusion and Restraint," in Tardiff, K., ed., *The Psychiatric Uses of Seclusion and Restraint*, pp. 1-9; p. 7.
47. See Szasz, T. S., *Insanity* and *Cruel Compassion.*
48. Lewis, C. S., "The humanitarian theory of punishment" [1949], in Lewis, C. S., Lewis, *God in the Dock,* pp. 287-294; pp. 292-293.
49. Moore, M. S., "Some myths about 'mental illness,'" *Archives of General Psychiatry*, 32: 1483-1497 (December), 1975; p. 1495.

Epilogue

1. Acton, J. E. E. D., "Liberty as the Reign of Conscience," *Essays in the Study and Writing of History*, vol. 3, pp. 489-491; p. 490.
2. Acton, J. E. E. D., "Letter to Mandell Creighton, April 5, 1887; Acton-Creighton Correspondence," in Acton, J. E. E. D., ibid., vol. 2, pp. 378-388; p. 383.

3. Chesterton, G. K., in *Illustrated London News,* April 19, 1930. Courtesy of Dale Ahlquist, President, American Chesterton Society.
4. Acton, J. E. E. D., "Antiquity," *Essays in the Study and Writing of History,* vol. 3, pp. 522-526; p. 523.
5. Szasz, T. S., *The Therapeutic State* and *Pharmacracy.*
6. Acton, J. E. E. D., "Democracy," *Essays in the Study and Writing of History,* vol. 3, pp. 549-557; pp. 556, 555.
7. Acton, J. E. E. D., "Letter to Johann Joseph Ignaz Dollinger, June 16, 1882," in ibid., pp. 665-674; p. 666. Dollinger was a prominent German theologian and, for many years, professor of church history and ecclesiastical law at the University of Munich. A learned man and devout Catholic, he was defrocked and excommunicated for his writings.
8. Ibid., p. 655.
9. Johnson, S., "Preface to the *Dictionary,*" in *Selected Writings,* p. 243.

Appendix I

1. Locke, J., *An Essay Concerning Human Understanding,* p. 9.
2. Acton, J. E. E. D., *Essays in the Study and Writing of History,* vol. 3, p. 550.
3. Szasz, T. S., *Pharmacracy.*
4. Loudon, I., *The Tragedy of Childbed Fever,* p. 59, emphasis added.
5. Quoted in Weissmann, G., "Puerperal priority," http://www.msu.edu/course/lbs/133/stillwell/puerperalp.html, emphasis added. See also Gordon A., *A Treatise on the Epidemic of Puerperal Fever of Aberdeen.*
6. Holmes, O. W., "The contagiousness of puerperal fever," *New England Quarterly Journal of Medicine and Surgery,* 1: 503-30, 1842.
7. Loudon, I., *The Tragedy of Childbed Fever,* p. 34.
8. Weissmann, G., "Puerperal priority," http://www.msu.edu/course/lbs/133/stillwell/puerperalp.html, emphasis added.
9. Ibid.
10. Benedek, I., *Semmelweis.*
11. Ibid.
12. Quoted in "Ignaz Phillip Semmelweis." http://clickit.go2net.com adclick?cid=187535&area=hm.dir.edu&site=hm&shape=exitpopup&keyword=embeddedexitpopup
13. See Powell, J., *The Triumph of Liberty.*
14. See Kendell, R. E., "The distinction between mental and physical illness" (Editorial), *British Journal of Psychiatry,* 178: 490-493, 2001.
15. Ibid., pp. 491, 492.
16. Leaning, J., "Health and human rights" (Editorial), *British Medical Journal,* 322: 1435-1436 (June 16), 2001. http://bmj.com/cgi/content/full/322/7300/1435
17. See for example Hebald, C., *The Heart Too Long Suppressed.*
18. White House Press Office, "White House Fact Sheet on Myths and Facts About Mental Illness," June 5, 1999. "Myths and Facts about Mental Illness," *New York Times,* June 7, 1999, Internet edition. See also, www.info@ariannaonline.com.
19. "Minerva," *British Medical Journal,* 322: 1132 (May 5), 2001.

Appendix II

1. Plautus, *Asinaria.* http://www.rjgeib.com/thoughts/killing/wolf.html.
2. Chekhov, A. P., *Ward No. 6,* in Szasz, T. S., ed., *The Age of Madness,* pp. 89-126; pp. 120-121.

3.   Szasz, T. S., *The Manufacture of Madness*, pp. 284, 288.
4.   Szasz, T. S., ed., *The Age of Madness*.
5.   Mill, J. S., "The Law of Lunacy" (Letter to the Editor of the *Daily News*, July 31, 1858), in *Collected Works of John Stuart Mill*, vol. 25, pp. 1198-1199.
6.   Talan, J., "20 years in psych facilities follow teen insanity plea," *Newsday*, August 20, 2001. http://www.newsday.com/news/health/ny-hstom192324915aug20.story
7.   Farley, M., "Mental illness by mandate," *Los Angeles Times*, February 10, 2000. http://www.latimes.com/news/nation/updates/lat_orphans000210.htm
8.   "Canadian orphans accept deal," *International Herald-Tribune*, July 3, 2001, p. 3.
9.   Reznick, R., "Judge decries patients' unjust 'imprisonment,'" *Ha'aretz*, November 9, 2000. http://www3.haaretz.co.il/eng/htmls/kat15_4.htm
10. Whittell, G., "War's forgotten man discovers himself," *Times* (London), August 25 2000, Internet edition.
11. Hundley, T., "'Last prisoner of WWII' looks for a memory: Held 56 years in Russia, Hungarian recalls little," *Chicago Tribune*, September 7, 2000, pp. 1 ff; and Internet edition.
12. Roberts, H., "A way forward for mental health in Ghana?" *The Lancet*, 357: 1859 (June 9), 2001.
13. Dougherty, J., "Testing the faith: Student sues college for psychiatric abuse, sent to mental ward after he objected to play depicting Jesus as homosexual," *WorldNetDaily*, January 5, 2001. http://www.scotsman.com/cfm/home/email_a_friend_part2.cfm © 2001 WorldNetDaily.com.
14. Leonnig, C. D., "Monitors Censure St. Elizabeths: Federal Funding Threatened After Patients Found Tied, Prone," *The Washington Post*, December 18, 2001. Internet edition.
15. For brief summaries, see http://www.epub.org.br/cm/n02/historia/lobotomy.htm; http://www.scc.net/~lkcmn/lobotomy/lobo/brief.html.
16. Alexander, G. J. and Scheflin, A. W., "Lobotomy," in Alexander, G. J. and Scheflin, A. W., *Law and Mental Disorder*, pp. 955-967; pp. 962-966.

Selected Bibliography

References to articles, reports, and other items appearing in journals, magazines, newspapers, and pamphlets are fully identified in the Notes. Books cited in the Notes only by author and title are identified more fully below.

Acton, J. E. E. D. *Essays in the Study and Writing of History*. Edited by J. Rufus Fears. 3 vols. Indianapolis: Liberty Classics, 1988.

Ahmed, P. I. and Plog, S. C., eds. *State Mental Hospitals: What Happens When They Close?* New York: Plenum, 1976.

Alexander, F. G. and Selesnick, S. T. *The History of Psychiatry: An Evaluation of Psychiatric Thought and Practice from Prehistoric Times to the Present*. New York: Harper & Row, 1966.

Alexander, G. J. and Scheflin, A. W. *Law and Mental Disorder*. Durham, NC: Carolina Academic Press, 1998.

American Psychiatric Association. *Diagnostic and Statistical Manual of MentalDisorders*. 3rd edition. Washington, DC: American Psychiatric Association, 1980.

Andreasen, N. C. *Brave New Brain: Conquering Mental Illness in the Era of the Genome*. New York: Oxford University Press, 2001.

Appelbaum, P. S. *Almost a Revolution: Mental Health Law and the Limits of Change*. New York: Oxford University Press, 1994.

Isaac, R. J. and Armat, V. C. *Madness in the Streets: How Psychiatry and the Law Abandoned the Mentally Ill*. New York: Free Press, 1990.

Auden, W. H. and Kronenberger, L., eds. *The Viking Book of Aphorisms: A Personal Selection*. New York: Dorset Pres, 1981.

Bartlett's Familiar Quotations. Sixteenth Edition. Edited by Justin Kaplan. Boston: Little, Brown & Co., 1992.

Batchelor, I. R. C. *Henderson and Gillespie's Textbook of Psychiatry*. Tenth Edition. London: Oxford University Press, 1969.

Bayer, R. *Homosexuality and American Psychiatry: The Politics of Diagnosis*. New York: Basic Books, 1981.

Benedek, I. *Semmelweis*. Budapest: Gondolat, 1980.

Black, H. C. *Black's Law Dictionary*. Revised Fourth Edition. St. Paul: West, 1968.

Blank, R. *Brain Policy: How the New Neuroscience Will Change Our Lives and Our Politics*. Washington, DC: Georgetown University Press, 1999.

Bleuler, E. *Dementia Praecox, or the Group of Schizophrenias* [1911]. Trans. by Joseph Zinkin. New York: International Universities Press, 1950.

Bleuler, E. *A Textbook of Psychiatry* [1924]. Translated by A. A. Brill. New York: Macmillan, 1944.

Bleuler, M. *The Schizophrenic Disorders: Long-Term Patient and Family Studies* [1972]. Translated by Siegfried M. Clemens. New Haven: Yale University Press, 1978.

Bloch, S. and Chodoff, P., eds. *Psychiatric Ethics*. Second Edition. Oxford: Oxford University Press, 1991.

Bynum, W. F., Porter, R., and Shepherd, M. eds. *The Anatomy of Madness: Essays in the History of Psychiatry*. 3 vols. London: Tavistock, 1985-1988.

Camus, A. *Resistance, Rebellion, Death*. Translated by Justin O'Brien. New York: Alfred A. Knopf, 1961.

Camus, A. *The Rebel: An Essay on Man in Revolt* [1951]. Translated by Anthony Bower. New York: Vintage Books, 1956.

Cannistraro, P. V. and Sullivan, B. R. *Il Duce's Other Woman*. New York: William Morrow, 1993.

Celine, L. F. *The Life and Work of Semmelweis* [1924], in Celine, L. F., *Mea Culpa & The Life and Work of Semmelweis*. Translated by Robert A. Parker. New York: Howard Fertig, 1979.

Chadwick, O. *Professor Lord Acton: The Regius Chair of Modern History at Cambridge, 1895-1902*. Grand Rapids, MI: Acton Institute, 1995.

Chekhov, A. P. *Seven Short Stories by Chekhov*. Translated by Barbara Makanowitzky. New York: Bantam Books, 1963.

Clare, A. *Psychiatry in Dissent: Controversial Issues in Thought and Practice*. London: Tavistock, 1976.

Coker, Richard J. *From Chaos to Coercion: Detention and the Control of Tuberculosis*. New York: St. Martin's Press, 2000.

Dante, A. *The Divine Comedy of Dante Alighieri*. New York: Oxford University Press, 1968.

Dante, A. *The Inferno*. Translated by John Ciardi. New York: Mentor, 1954.

Davis, D. B. *The Problem of Slavery in Western Culture*. Ithaca, NY: Cornell University Press, 1966.

Davis, D. B. *The Problem of Slavery in the Age of Revolution, 1770-1823*. Ithaca, NY: Cornell University Press, 1975.

Davis, D. B. *Slavery and Human Progress*. New York, Oxford University Press, 1984.

Dennis, D. L. and Monahan, J., eds. *Coercion and Aggressive Community Treatment: A New Frontier in Mental Health Law*. New York: Plenum, 1996.

Deutsch, A. *The Shame of the States*. New York: Harcourt, Brace and Company, 1948.

Deutsch, A. *The Mentally Ill in America: A History of Their Care and Treatment from Colonial Times*. 2nd ed. New York: Columbia University Press, 1952.

Dolnick, E. *Madness on the Couch: Blaming the Victim in the Heyday of Psychoanalysis*. New York, Simon & Schuster, 1998.

Dostoyevski, F. *Notes from Underground* [1864]. Translated by Jessie Coulson. Harmondsworth, UK: Penguin, 1972.

Ellison, R. *Invisible Man* [1952]. New York: Modern Library, 1994.

Encyclopaedia Britannica. 16th Edition. Chicago: Encyclopaedia Britannica, 1973.

Fehrenbacher, Don E. *The Dred Scott Case: Its Significance in American Law and Politics.* New York: Oxford University Press, 1978.

Feynman, R. P. *"What Do You Care What Other People Think?": Further Adventures of a Curious Character.* New York: Bantam Books, 1989.

Feynman, R. P. *The Pleasure of Finding Things Out: The Best Short Works of Richard P. Feynman.* Edited by Jeffrey Robbins. Cambridge: Perseus Publishing, 1999.

Finkelman, P. *Slavery and the Founders: Race and Liberty in the Age of Jefferson.* Armonk, NY: M. E. Sharpe, 1996.

Finkelman, P., ed. *His Soul Goes Marching On: Responses to John Brown and the Harpers Ferry Raid.* Charlottesville: University of Virginia Press, 1995.

Foley, H. A. and Sharfstein, S. S. *Madness and Government: Who Cares for the Mentally Ill?* Washington, DC: American Psychiatric Press, 1983.

Foner, P. S., ed. *The Life and Major Writings of Thomas Paine.* Secaucus, NJ: Citadel Press, 1974.

Geller, J, L. and Harris, M., eds. *Women of the Asylum: Voices from Behind the Walls, 1840-1945.* New York: Doubleday Anchor, 1994.

Gelman, S. *Medicating Schizophrenia: A History.* New Brunswick, NJ: Rutgers University Press, 1999.

Gijswijt-Hofstra, M. and Porter, R., eds. *Cultures of Psychiatry and Mental Health Care in Postwar Britain and the Netherlands.* Amsterdam, NL: Editions Rodopi, 1998.

Goffman, E. *Asylums: Essays on the Social Situation of Mental Patients and Other Inmates.* Garden City, N. Y.: Doubleday Anchor, 1961.

Goffman, E. *Stigma: Notes on the Management of Spoiled Identity.* Englewood Cliffs, NJ: Prentice-Hall, 1963.

Gordon A. *A Treatise on the Epidemic of Puerperal Fever of Aberdeen.* London: G. G. & J. Robinson, 1795.

Gordon, R. *Great Medical Disasters.* New York: Stein and Day, 1983.

Gosden, R. *Punishing the Patient: How Psychiatrists Misunderstand and Mistreat Schizophrenia.* Melbourne, Australia: Scribe Publications, 2001.

Gostin, L. O. *Public Health Law: Power, Duty, Restraint.* Berkeley and Los Angeles: University of California Press, 2000.

Grasset, J. *The Semi-Insane and the Semi-Responsible. (Demifous et Demiresponsable.)* Translated by Smith Ely Jelliffe. New York: Funk and Wagnalls, 1907.

Hall, J. K., et al., eds. *One Hundred Years of American Psychiatry* (For the American Psychiatric Association). New York: Columbia University Press, 1944.

Hayek, F. A. *The Constitution of Liberty.* Chicago: University of Chicago Press, 1960.

Healy, D. *The Antidepressant Era.* Cambridge: Harvard University Press, 1998.

Hebald, C. *The Heart Too Long Suppressed: A Chronicle of Mental Illness.* Boston: Northeastern University Press, 2001.

Hill, R. G. *The Total Abolition of Personal Restraint in the Treatment of the Insane: A Lecture on the Management of Lunatic Asylums, and the Treat-*

ment of the Insane. London: Simpkin, Marshall & Co, 1839. Facsimile reprint. New York: Arno Press, 1976.

Hobson, J. A. and Leonard, J. *Out of Its Mind: Psychiatry in Crisis, A Call for Reform.* Cambridge, MA: Perseus Publishing, 2001.

Hoffman, A. *Inventing Mark Twain: The Lives of Samuel Langhorne Clemens.* New York: William Morrow, 1997.

Holland, W. W., Detels, R., and Knox, G., eds. *Oxford Textbook of Public Health.* 2nd ed. 2 vols. New York: Oxford University Press, 1991.

Hunter, R. and Macalpine, I., eds. *Three Hundred Years of Psychiatry, 1535-1860: A History Presented in Selected English Texts.* London: Oxford University Press, 1963.

Intellectual Freedom Manual. Fifth edition. Chicago: American Library Association, 1996.

Isaac, R. J. and Armat, V. C. *Madness in the Streets: How Psychiatry and the Law Abandoned the Mentally Ill.* New York: Free Press, 1990.

Isaac, R. J. and Isaac, E. *The Coercive Utopians: Social Deception by America's Power Players.* Chicago: Regnery, 1983.

Jamison, K. R. *An Unquiet Mind: A Memoir of Mood* and *Madness.* New York: Knopf, 1995.

Jamison, K. R. *Night Falls Fast: Understanding Suicide.* New York: Knopf, 1999.

Jaspers, K. *General Psychopathology* [1913, 1946]. Seventh Edition. Translated by J. Hoenig and M. W. Hamilton. Chicago: University of Chicago Press, 1963.

Johnson, A. B. *Out of Bedlam: The Truth About Deinstitutionalization.* New York: Basic Books, 1990.

Johnson, S. *Johnson's Dictionary: A Modern Selection* [1755]. Edited by E. L. McAdam, Jr. and George Milne. New York: Pantheon, 1963.

Johnson, S. *Selected Writings.* Edited by Patrick Cruttwell. London: Penguin, 1986.

Johnstone, L. *Users and Abusers of Psychiatry.* Second Edition. London: Routledge, 2000.

Kaplan, H. I. and Sadock, B. J. *Kaplan and Sadock's Synopsis of Psychiatry, Behavioral Sciences/Clinical Psychiatry.* Eighth edition. Philadelphia: Lippincott, Williams & Wlkins, 1998.

Kimball, R. *Experiments Against Reality: The Fate of Culture in the Postmodern World.* Chicago: Ivan R. Dee, 2000.

Kirk, R. *Lord Acton on Revolution.* Grand Rapids, MI: Acton Institute, 1994.

Kolb, L. C. *Noyes' Modern Clinical Psychiatry.* Seventh Edition. Philadelphia: W. B. Saunders, 1968.

Kraditor, A. S. *Means and Ends in American Abolitionism: Garrison and His Critics on Strategy and Tactics, 1834-1850.* New York: Random House, 1969.

Kraepelin, E. *Lectures on Clinical Psychiatry.* A Facsimile of the 1904 Edition. Translated by Thomas Johnstone. New York: Hafner, 1968.

Kraepelin, E. *One Hundred Years of Psychiatry* [1917]. Translated by Wade Baskin. New York: Philosophical Library, 1962.

Krafft-Ebing, R. *Psychopathia Sexualis, with Special Reference to the*

Antipathic Sexual Instinct: A Medico-Forensic Study [1886/1906]. Authorized English adaptation of the twelfth German edition by F. J. Rebman. Revised edition. Brooklyn, NY: Physicians and Surgeons Book Company, 1931.

Kroger, L. *Black Slaveowners: Free Black Slave Masters in South Carolina, 1790-1860.* Columbia, SC: University of South Carolina Press, 1985.

La Fond, John Q. And Mary L. Durham. *Back to the Asylum: The Future of Mental Health Law and Policy in the United States.* New York: Oxford University Press, 1992.

Leichter, H. M. *Free to be Foolish: Politics and Health Promotion in the United States and Great Britain.* Princeton: Princeton University Press, 1991.

Lewis, C. S. *God in the Dock: Essays on Theology and Ethics.* Edited by Walter Hooper. Grand Rapids, MI: William B. Eerdmans, 1970.

Lion, J. and Reid, W. H. *Assaults Within Psychiatric Facilities.* New York: Grune & Stratton, 1983.

Loudon, I. Irvine. *The Tragedy of Childbed Fever.* Oxford: Oxford University Press, 2000.

Luhrmann, T. M. *Of Two Minds: The Growing Disorder in American Psychiatry.* New York: Knopf, 2000.

Mabee, C. *Black Freedom: The Nonviolent Abolitionists from 1830 Through the Civil War.* New York: Macmillan, 1970.

Macmillan Book of Proverbs, Maxims, and Famous Phrases, The. Edited by B. Stevenson. New York: Macmillan, 1948.

Magnet, M. *The Dream and the Nigthmare: The Sixties' Legacy to the Underclass* [1993]. San Francisco: Encounter Books, 2000.

Maine, H. S. *Ancient Law: Its Connection With the Early History of Society, and Its Relation to Modern Ideas* [1864], Foreword by Lawrence Rosen. Tucson: University of Arizona Press, 1986.

Margolis, H. *Paradigms & Barriers: How Habits of Mind Govern Scientific Beliefs.* Chicago: University of Chicago Press, 1993.

Marks, J. *The Search for the "Manchurian Candidate": The CIA and Mind Control.* New York: Times Books, 1979.

Martindale, D. and Martindale E. *Psychiatry and the Law: The Crusade Against Involuntary Hospitalization.* St. Paul, MN: Windflower Publishing Co., 1973.

McElrath, D., Holland, J., White, W., and S. Katzman. *Lord Action, The Decisive Decade, 1864-1874: Essays and Documents,* Louvain, Belgium: Publications Universitaires de Louvain, 1970.

McPherson, James M. *Battle Cry of Freedom: The Civil War Era.* New York: Oxford, 1988.

Maudsley, H. *Responsibility in Mental Disease.* 4th edition. London: Kegan Paul, Trench & Co., 1885.

Mayer, H. *All on Fire: William Lloyd Garrison and the Abolition of Slavery.* New York: St. Martin's Press, 1998.

Menninger, K. *The Vital Balance: The Life Process in Mental Health and Illness.* New York: Viking, 1963.

Menninger, K. *The Crime of Punishment.* New York: Viking, 1968.

Menninger, R. W. and Nemiah, J. C., eds. *American Psychiatry After World War*

II (1944-1994). Washington, DC: American Psychiatric Press, 2000.

Mill, J. S. *Collected Works of John Stuart Mill.* Edited by Ann P. Robson and John M. Robson. Toronto: University of Toronto Press, 1986.

Morris, T. D. *Southern Slavery and the Law, 1619-1860.* Chapel Hill, NC: The University of North Carolina Press, 1996.

Noonan J. T., Jr. *Persons and Masks of the Law.* New York: Farrar, Straus and Giroux, 1976.

Parry-Jones, W. Ll. *The Trade in Lunacy: A Study of Private Madhouses in England in the Eighteenth and Nineteenth Centuries.* London: Routledge & Kegan Paul, 1976.

Pence, G. E. *Classic Cases in Medical Ethics: Accounts of Cases that Have Shaped Medical Ethics, with Philosophical, Legal, and Historical Backgrounds.* Boston: McGraw-Hill, 1990.

Pinard, G.-F. and Pagani, L., eds. *Clinical Assessment of Dangerousness: Empirical Contributions.* New York: Cambridge University Press, 2000.

Powell, J. *The Triumph of Liberty: A 2,000-Year History, Told Through the Lives of Freedom's Greatest Champions.* New York: Free Press, 2000.

Revel, J.-F. *The Totalitarian Temptation.* Translated by David Hapgood. Garden City, NY: Doubleday, 1977.

Ridgely, M. S., Borum, R., and Petrila, J. *The Effectiveness of Involuntary Outpatient Treatment: Empirical Evidence and the Experience of Eight States.* Santa Monica, CA: Rand Corporation, 2001.

Robitscher, J. *The Powers of Psychiatry.* Boston: Houghton Mifflin, 1980.

Ross, C. and Pam, A. *Pseudoscience in Biological Psychiatry: Blaming the Body.* New York: Wiley, 1994.

Rothman, D. J. *The Discovery of the Asylum: Social Order and Disorder in the New Republic.* Boston: Little, Brown, 1971.

Rush, B. *Autobiography of Benjamin Rush: His "Travels through Life" together with His "Commonplace Book for 1789-1812."* Edited by G. W. Corner. Princeton: Princeton University Press, 1948.

Rush, B. *Letters of Benjamin Rush.* Edited by L. H. Butterfield. 2 vols. Princeton: Princeton University Press, 1951.

Rush, B. *Medical Inquiries and Observations upon the Diseases of the Mind* (1812). New York: Macmillan-Hafner Press, 1962.

Satel, S. *PC, M.D.: How Political Correctness is Corrupting Medicine.* New York: Basic Books, 2000.

Sayce, L. *From Psychiatric Patient to Citizen: Overcoming Discrimination and Social Exclusion.* New York: St. Martin's Press, 2000.

Schiller, L. and Bennett, A. *The Quiet Room: A Journey Out of the Torment of Madness.* New York: Warner Books, 1977.

Scull, A., MacKenzie, C., and Hervey, N. *Masters of Bedlam: The Transformation of the Mad-Doctoring Trade.* Princeton: Princeton University Press, 1996.

Secunda, V. *When Madness Comes Home: Help and Hope for the Children, Siblings, and Partners of the Mentally Ill.* New York: Hyperion, 1997.

Simon, R. I. *Concise Guide to Psychiatry and the Law for Clinicians.* Third edition. Washington, DC: American Psychiatric Press, 2001.

Simmons, A. J. *Justification and Legitimacy: Essays on Rights and Obliga-tions*. Cambridge: Cambridge University Press, 2001.

Skultans, V. *Madness and Morals: Ideas on Insanity in the Nineteenth Century*. London: Routledge & Kedgan Paul, 1975.

Stefan, S. *Unequal Rights: Discrimination Against People With Mental Dis-abilities and the Americans with Disabilities Act*. Washington, DC: Ameri-can Psychological Association, 2001.

Stein, L. I. and Santos, A. B. *Assertive Community Treatment of Persons with Severe Mental Illness*. New York: Norton: 1998.

Stolle, D. P., Winick, B. J., and Wexler, D. B. *Practicing Therapeutic Jurispru-dence: Law as a Helping Profession*. Durham, NC: Carolina Academic Press, 2000.

Stone, A. A. *Law, Psychiatry and Morality*. Washington, DC: American Psychi-atric Press, 1985.

Szasz, T. S. *Anti-Freud: Karl Kraus's Criticism of Psychoanalysis and Psychia-try* [1976]. Syracuse: Syracuse University Press, 1990.

Szasz, T. S. *Ceremonial Chemistry: The Ritual Persecution of Drugs, Addicts, and Pushers* [1976]. Revised edition. Holmes Beach, FL: Learning Pub-lications, 1985.

Szasz, T. S. *Cruel Compassion: The Psychiatric Control of Society's Unwanted* [1994]. Syracuse: Syracuse University Press, 1998.

Szasz, T. S. *The Ethics of Psychoanalysis: The Theory and Method of Autono-mous Psychotherapy* [1965]. With a new preface. Syracuse: Syracuse University Press, 1988.

Szasz, T. S. *Fatal Freedom: The Ethics and Politics of Suicide*. Westport, CT: Praeger, 1999.

Szasz, T. S. *Ideology and Insanity: Essays on the Psychiatric Dehumanization of Man* [1970]. Syracuse: Syracuse University Press, 1991.

Szasz, T. S. *Insanity: The Idea and Its Consequences* [1987]. Syracuse: Syra-cuse University Press, 1997.

Szasz, T. S. *Law, Liberty, and Psychiatry: An Inquiry Into the Social Uses of Mental Health Practices* [1963]. Syracuse: Syracuse University Press, 1989.

Szasz, T. S. *A Lexicon of Lunacy: Metaphoric Malady, Moral Responsibility, and Psychiatry*. New Brunswick, NJ: Transaction Publishers, 1993.

Szasz, T. S. *The Manufacture of Madness: A Comparative Study of the Inquisi-tion and the Mental Health Movement* [1970]. With a new preface. Syra-cuse: Syracuse University Press, 1997.

Szasz, T. S. *The Meaning of Mind: Language, Morality, and Neuroscience*. New York: Praeger, 1996.

Szasz, T. S. *The Myth of Mental Illness: Foundations of a Theory of Personal Conduct* [1961]. Revised edition. New York: HarperCollins, 1974.

Szasz, T. S., *The Myth of Psychotherapy: Mental Healing as Religion, Rhetoric, and Repression* [1978]. Syracuse: Syracuse University Press, 1988.

Szasz, T. S. *Our Right to Drugs: The Case for a Free Market*. Westport, CT: Praeger, 1992.

Szasz, T. S. *Pharmacracy: Medicine and Politics in America*. Westport, CT: Praeger, 2001.

Szasz, T. S. *Psychiatric Justice* [1965]. With a new preface. Syracuse: Syracuse University Press, 1988.

Szasz, T. S. *Psychiatric Slavery: When Confinement and Coercion Masquerade as Cure* [1977]. Syracuse: Syracuse University Press, 1998.

Szasz, T. S. *The Second Sin.* Garden City, NY: Doubleday Anchor, 1973.

Szasz, T. S. *Sex By Prescription* [1980]. Syracuse: Syracuse University Press, 1990.

Szasz, T .S. *The Theology of Medicine: The Political-Philosophical Foundations of Medical Ethics* [1977]. With a new preface. Syracuse: Syracuse University Press, 1988.

Szasz, T. S. *The Therapeutic State: Psychiatry in the Mirror of Current Events.* Buffalo: Prometheus Books, 1984.

Szasz, T. S. *The Untamed Tongue: A Dissenting Dictionary.* LaSalle, IL: Open Court, 1990.

Szasz, T. S., ed. *The Age of Madness: A History of Involuntary Mental Hospitalization Presented in Selected Texts.* Garden City, NY: Doubleday Anchor, 1973.

Union Pacific Railway Co. v. Botsford, 141 U.S. 250, 251.

Tannsjo, T. *Coercive Care: The Ethics of Choice in Health and Medicine.* London: Routledge, 1999.

Tardiff, K., ed. *Psychiatric Uses of Seclusion and Restraint.* Washington, DC: American Psychiatric Press, 1984.

Templeton, K. S. Jr., ed. *The Politicization of Society.* Indianapolis, IN: Liberty Press, 1979.

Torrey, E. F., ed. *Ethical Issues in Medicine: The Role of the Physician in Today's Society.* Boston: Little, Brown and Company, 1968.

Torrey, E. F. *Nowhere To Go: The Tragic Odyssey of the Homeless Mentally Ill .* New York: Harper & Row, 1988.

Torrey, E. F., et al. *Criminalizing the Seriously Mentally Ill: The Abuse of Jails as Mental Hospitals.* Washington, DC: The National Alliance for the Mentally Ill and Public Citizen's Health Research Group, 1992.

Ulrich, L. P. *The Patient Self-Determination Act: Meeting the Challenges in Patient Care.* Washington, DC: Georgetown University Press, 1999.

Van Gogh, V. *Dear Theo: The Autobiography of Vincent Van Gogh* [1937]. Edited by Irving Stone. New York: Signet/New American Library, 1969.

Van Gogh, V., *The Complete Letters of Vincent Van Gogh, With Reproductions of All the Drawings in the Correspondence.* 3 Vols. Boston: New York Graphics Society, 1958.

Wear, A., ed. *Medicine in Society: Historical Essays.* Cambridge: Cambridge University Press, 1992.

Wexler, D. B. and Winick, B. J., eds., *Essays in Therapeutic Jurisprudence.* Durham, NC: Carolina Academic Press, 1991.

Wexler, D. B. and Winick, B. J., eds., *Law in a Therapeutic Key: Developments in Therapeutic Jurisprudence.* Durham, NC: Carolina Academic Press, 1996.

Whitehead, A. N. *Adventures of Ideas* [1933]. New York: Free Press, 1961.

Whitten, D. O. *Andrew Durnford: A Black Sugar Planter in the Antebellum South*. New Brunswick, NJ: Transaction Publishers, 1995.

Wiethoff, W. E. *A Peculiar Humanism: The Judicial Advocacy of Slavery in High Courts of the Old South, 1820-1850*. Athens, GA: University of Georgia Press, 1996.

Winchester, S. *The Professor and the Madman: A Tale of Murder, Insanity, and the Making of the Oxford English Dictionary*. New York: HarperCollins, 1998.

Winick, B. J. *The Right to Refuse Mental Health Treatment*. Washington, DC: American Psychological Association, 1997.

Winick, B. J., *Therapeutic Jurisprudence Applied : Essays on Mental Health Law*. Durham, NC: Carolina Academic Press, 1997.

Zilboorg, G. and Henry, G. *A History of Medical Psychology*. New York: Norton, 1941.

Index

Printed in the United States
by Baker & Taylor Publisher Services